Children of Poverty

Studies and Dissertations on
the Effects of Single Parenthood,
the Feminization of Poverty,
and Homelessness

Stuart Bruchey
UNIVERSITY OF MAINE
General Editor

A Garland Series

Doped Up, Knocked Up, and ... Locked Up?

The Criminal Prosecution of Women Who Use Drugs During Pregnancy

Valerie Green

Garland Publishing, Inc.
New York & London
1993

Library of Congress Cataloging-in-Publication Data

Green, Valerie, 1970–
    Doped up, knocked up, and . . . locked up? : the criminal prosecution of women who
use drugs during pregnancy / Valerie Green.
        p. cm. — (Children of poverty)
    Includes bibliographical references.
    ISBN 0–8153–1125–7 (alk. paper)
    1. Narcotic laws—United States. 2. Prosecution—United States. 3. Drug abuse in
pregnancy—United States. 4. Fetus—Effects of drugs on.   I. Title. II. Series.
KF3890.G74 1993
364.1'77—dc20   92–35296
                                                                                  CIP

Printed on acid-free, 250-year-life paper
Manufactured in the United States of America

For my parents for their unending love and support

-veg

Contents

Preface

This project began almost exactly two years ago at the onset of my senior year at Barnard College. When I first started thinking about my senior thesis I had no idea that it could be so rewarding and so enlightening.

My topic, the prosecution of women who use drugs during pregnancy, first came to me during a discussion with my adviser about Katha Pollitt's article, "A New Assault on Feminism," that appeared in *The Nation* in March, 1990. I had been looking for a way to write about women and social policy, so when I read about the incredible injustice and shortsightedness of these punitive measures I was spurred on to learn more about the women whose lives are discussed in these pages.

Because the original research is over one and one half years old, many of the women's lives examined here have changed, some for the better, others for the worse. I sometimes find it hard to believe that the legal system managed to review these cases so quickly, but it did. I have tried to update the information to incorporate the changes here.

My hope is that my data will soon be out of date and the new data will reveal that drug use among pregnant women is declining, not rising; that high quality pre-natal care is accessible to all women; that drug treatment programs have adjusted to accommodate the needs of pregnant drug addicts; and that the crusade to restrict women's autonomy and privacy has died out. My idealism reveals my age.

In closing, I would like to thank Garland Publishing, Inc. for giving me this thrill and for enabling me to share this with others.

Valerie Green
October 1, 1992

Acknowledgments

Of course, I cannot take all the credit for this thesis. Many wonderful people (and places) have helped me along the way.

Leslie, I thank you for your inspiration, your guidance, your criticism and your witticism.

Thank you Phyllis Segal for taking the time to read this thesis and to bolster my confidence; Judy Russell for reading with an approving eye; Sue Kerr for your unending patience during our senior year; Chris Grillo for your "finishing" touches; and Claudia Hirsch for being my editor and, more essentially, my soul sister.

Barnard College, who would ever have thought you could push me so hard.

To my toughest critic and most encouraging partner in crime, Matthew, I owe great gratitude for commas, periods, and love.

For my family, Melissa, Mom, Dad, you know that were it not for the unique combination of love that you provide me, I would not have taken this step. Thank you.

Introduction

The number of babies born addicted to drugs has risen dramatically in recent years. Many experts estimate that in 1989 alone as many as 375,000 babies were exposed to drugs before they were born.[1] According to the National Association for Perinatal Addiction Research and Education (NAPARE), pre-natal exposure to controlled substances such as marijuana, cocaine, crack cocaine, heroin, PCP, and amphetamines can lead to pre-natal strokes, premature or even still birth, tremors, deficient motor reflexes, and learning disabilities if the child survives infancy.[2] These drug-babies require more intensive and longer hospital stays than babies born drug-free.

The reason for the increase in babies born addicted to or exposed to controlled substances is the rise in drug use among pregnant women. A survey of thirty-six hospitals across the United States conducted by NAPARE discovered that 11 percent of the women who gave birth in these hospitals had used illegal drugs (marijuana, cocaine, PCP, heroin, amphetamines) during their pregnancies. This means that more than one in ten women uses drugs during pregnancy.

Society is confronted with a complex problem: who will be held responsible for the growing number of babies born addicted to drugs? This thesis will address the issue of the prosecution of women who use drugs during pregnancy. Holding women solely responsible for the condition of their babies at birth, some states have attempted to prosecute women for using drugs during pregnancy.

In light of the growing crisis, the prosecution of women is an understandable reaction: Quite simply, there is only one way for a fetus to be exposed to drugs: through the umbilical cord. So, on some (physiological) level, pregnant women are directly responsible for pre-natal drug exposure. However, society's initial reaction, the prosecution of pregnant drug users, cannot solve the problem; it cannot protect fetuses from exposure to drugs through the umbilical cord.

The criminal prosecution of women who use drugs during pregnancy is an incomplete and misdirected effort at eliminating drug use among pregnant women of all races and economic classes and wiping out the crisis of drug babies. The issue at hand is at least two-dimensional; one aspect is the overwhelming number of babies being born exposed to controlled substances. Understandably, society has reacted with compassion and sympathy for these infants; the criminal prosecution of their mothers has been conceived of as a way to protect these babies from further harm. It can also be seen as a preventive measure; prosecutors hope that by making it a crime to give birth to a baby who tests positive for a controlled substance women will be deterred from using drugs during pregnancy.

So far, it has not worked. The number of women using drugs during pregnancy is on the rise; and this is the second dimension of the problem. Many of the women who use drugs during pregnancy, and especially those who are being prosecuted, are not only unable to receive treatment for their drug addictions and dependencies, but also are without proper pre-natal care. These two problems must be addressed together if the desired result is healthy, drug free babies; in the same way that a mother's addiction and poor health can damage her fetus, her good health and freedom from addiction can improve her fetus' chance of being born and remaining healthy.

In March 1990 an article printed in *The Nation* stated that one-fifth of the pregnant women in this country receive no pre-natal care at all.[3] This means that 20% of the pregnant women in this country do not interact with health care professionals until they actually give birth; by that time it is too late to *educate* pregnant women about the harmful effects drugs can have on a developing fetus, to refer them to treatment programs if necessary, and to monitor the development of the fetus. There are many reasons that such a startling number of women can not benefit from pre-natal care in this country; they range from poverty to a lack of facilities. These issues will be addressed in Chapter 3 as they effect the companion crises of drug babies and the criminal prosecution of their mothers.

The question of drug addiction and treatment will also be addressed as an underlying cause of this issue. As access to pre-natal care is limited so, too, is access to drug treatment. Most drug treatment programs refuse, point blank, to admit pregnant women claiming that they are either not equipped to accommodate the special needs of pregnant women (because they can not provide pre-natal care or day-care for small children) or are unwilling to accept the responsibility for the effect of drug rehabilitation on the fetus (even though withdrawal is only *potentially* harmful for fetuses).[4] Recently, new efforts have been made to design drug treatment facilities to meet these special needs of women addicts, but such pilot programs are expensive and not yet adequate to meet the demands of the growing crisis. (These new facilities will be discussed in Chapter 3 as part of the solution.)

The criminalization of women's behavior during pregnancy presents legal as well as social problems. As it ignores the underlying causes of drug use among pregnant women, so too, it disregards the effect that such a social policy could have on the relationship between a woman and her fetus, and the potential repercussions for women's rights. Chapter 1 will provide a history of the fetus in the law and the development of the doctrine of privacy by the Supreme Court. The legal relationship of parents to their children[5] will also be examined. Because all of the legal precedents indicate that women's rights should take precedence over fetal rights, tracing the evolution of the status of the fetus in the law, from an entity considered solely as a part of its mother to an entity entitled to some protection by the state, can help to distill the issues surrounding fetal rights. The fetus has been granted increasing legal protection over the past two hundred years. Its status has been affected by ever-changing political agendas and is a major point of contention in the debate over the criminal prosecution of women who use drugs during pregnancy.

Chapter 2 will document the development of the methods used by district attorneys around the country in order to establish standards of societally acceptable behavior during pregnancy. The earliest cases of criminal prosecution of women who use drugs during pregnancy were unsuccessful. At first, courts were unwilling to punish women for actions that were never intended to be considered crimes under child abuse and neglect laws, and drug trafficking statutes; fetuses were simply never intended to be protected under these statutes at the time that they were enacted. Over the last four or five years, prosecutors have developed increasingly meticulous and ingenious methods of prosecuting women who use drugs during pregnancy in order to overcome these defeats. Chapter 2 will examine the evolution of these techniques. The second chapter will also address issues of race and class as they affect decisions about the who's and how's of prosecuting women for drug use during pregnancy.

Medical professionals and judges can play roles in the criminal prosecution of drug-using pregnant women; they can either aid or hinder prosecutors in their attempts to put pregnant drug addicts behind bars. Their involvement will be examined in Chapter 2, as well.

It is as a result of the increasing appeal of prosecuting, rather than helping, these women that many feminists and civil libertarians fear the widespread acceptance of the criminal prosecution of women who use drugs during pregnancy into current law. It could have potentially far-reaching implications for the rights of women as members of this society. Women's rights to privacy and bodily integrity could be lost in a society that is willing to protect the fetus at the expense of its mother's freedom rather than work toward a complete solution to the problem.

Chapter 3 will examine the underlying causes of the crisis brought on by drug use among pregnant women. It will also examine the underlying motivations behind the criminal prosecution of these women. Because the root of the problem is not the behavior of women during pregnancy in general, the solution must not exclude women; women, too, must benefit from any comprehensive plan to alleviate this crisis. Rather than alienating pregnant women from their fetuses and subjecting them to stricter standards of behavior than other individuals, society should work to protect women from the abuses of poverty and drug addiction with the same enthusiasm that it exhibits when championing the rights of the fetus.

If the criminal prosecution of women who use drugs during pregnancy becomes the dominant method of combating the rise in infants born exposed to controlled substances both women and their babies will suffer. The rights of women to autonomy will be subjugated to the rights of the fetus to be born in good health. The societal problems of poverty, inadequate pre-natal care and drug treatment for pregnant women will be left unaddressed.

NOTES

1 "A First: National Hospital Incidence Survey," NAPARE *Update* October 1988.

2 Susan LaCroix, "Jailing Mothers for Drug Abuse," *The Nation*, 1 May 1989, p. 585.

3 Katha Pollitt, "A New Assault on Feminism," *The Nation*, 26 March 1990, p. 410.

4 Michael Freitag, "Hospital Defends Limiting of Drug Program," *New York Times*, 12 October 1989, sec. II, p. 9. "Suit Seeks Drug Treatment for Pregnant Women," *New York Times*, 10 December 1989, p. 62.

5 Despite the fact that fetuses are not yet "children," the legal nature of this relationship merits discussion. The question of whether an unborn fetus can be protected by laws that were designed to protect "children" is central to the debate over whether a woman can be held liable for damage suffered by her fetus. See Chapter 1 supra.

Doped Up, Knocked Up, and . . . Locked Up?

I

The Fetus and the Woman in Law:
a History

"The legal status that society chooses to confer upon the fetus is dependent upon the goals being pursued and the effect of such status on competing values."[1] Thus the legal status of the fetus in America has changed over the past two hundred years to fit the ever-changing political agenda. In common law, tort law, inheritance law, and criminal law, the fetus has become an entity entitled to protection under the law and to compensation for damages. However, the legal status of the fetus is at best unclear: The Supreme Court has refused to grant constitutional protection under the Fourteenth Amendment to the fetus, yet today many state statutes protect the fetus. A review of the fetus in the law and the evolution of the rights of privacy can help to explain the legal controversy surrounding the criminal prosecution of women who use drugs during pregnancy.

Historically, the fetus has been considered to be part of its mother and has enjoyed very few rights as a separate entity. However, in some specific circumstances fetal rights have been recognized. Courts have granted retroactive legal personhood to fetuses in order to protect their rights *after* they are born. Traditionally, fetal rights were contingent on live birth; that is, once a

3

fetus is born alive, courts are willing to award rights and
protections as recognition that the child was once a fetus
in utero. To reiterate, a fetus who had suffered injury
while in utero was able to bring suit and recover for
those damages only *after* it was born alive.

In the landmark 1973 decision *Roe v Wade*, the
Supreme Court concluded that,"the unborn have never
been recognized in the law as persons in the whole
sense."[2] The Court also explained that traditionally legal
rights were granted to the fetus "[only] in narrowly
defined situations and [only] when the rights [were]
contingent upon live birth."[3]

The fetus, according to the Supreme Court, is not
protected by the 14th Amendment as a "person," but
courts have become more willing to grant the fetus
protection   under   "substantive   non-fourteenth
Amendment law," like tort law and child abuse and
neglect laws, since the *Roe* decision established that a
state interest in the health of the fetus certainly does
exist.decision that can be based on biology.[4]

THE FETUS AS A PART OF THE WOMAN:
THE TRADITION

For most of legal history, the fetus, qua fetus, was
granted legal protection, precisely because it was
considered to be a part of its mother. Courts intended to
protect the interest of born persons, whether it was a
newborn infant or its parents. Laws that granted rights
to a fetus were intended to protect newborns (recently
fetuses) as well as parents.   When fetuses were
regognized in inheritance law, common law, tort law,
and criminal law it was only on the condition that the

fetus, which is while geststing still only a part of its mother, would later become a person in its own right. The following precedents illustrate that the fetus was not entitled to protection and did not have rights; its position as a part of its mother, and its potential to be born alive were the only ways for the fetus to gain legal recognition.

Common Law and Inheritance Law

In common law, the destruction of a fetus was not considered a homicide. It was illegal to harm a fetus by harming the mother only if the fetus was born alive and then died. Women in the past have been able to recover damages for "their own injuries caused by miscarriage" but not " for the loss of the child. These cases reflect the court's desire to allow parents to recover damages for their loss.[5] There are cases dating from 1797 that hold that a state must be able to show "actual physical independence of a [fetus] to sustain a conviction for a homicide."[6]

The fetus was recognized very early in inheritance and property laws. In many inhertance disputes[7] courts found on behalf of the fetus in order to protect the will of the testator (a born persdon), and to enable a child (once it was born) to benefit. It was not in order to establish the fetus as a legal person.

Tort Law

Before 1946, courts would not recognize tort claims brought by infants (or rather, by someone else on behalf of a fetus) for injuries inflicted before birth. In 1884, a suit was brought against the town of Northampton,

Massachusetts for damages suffered by a pregnant woman when she tripped on a poorly constructed sidewalk. The decision in the case, *Dietrich v Inhabitants of Northampton* ,[8] which denied recovery for damages to a 4-5 month old fetus, went unchallenged as the rule regarding pre-natal injury until 1946.

In 1946, tortious injury was inflicted by two physicians upon a viable fetus. For the first time ever, a court recognized the right of a child to sue for damages inflicted *in utero*. This state court, however, still required that the injury be inflicted after viability, which is the point at which a fetus can exist, on its own, outside its mother.[9] So, the prerequisite for a fetus gaining legal status is to establish, by meeting the court defined standards of viability, its potential for independance from its mother. The decision in this case, *Bombrest v Kotz* ,[10] limited recovery to fetuses injured after viability, and then only if the fetus was subsequently born alive. In 1949, *Verkennes v Corniea*[11] extended the rule: Courts were willing to entertain wrongful death suits brought on behalf of stillborn fetuses, as well. Allowances for these suits were made in order to compensate survivors for the loss of a family member due to injury that could have been prevented. Live birth was a requirement at one point but it is no longer, because its effect was to punish someone for maiming a fetus subsequently born, but not for killing it.[12] These suits, which were aimed at the recovery of damages, were brought against third parties, like doctors or employers, rather than against mothers. Wrongful death claims were intended to compensate the parents for the loss of their child, as well as to help cover medical costs and burial charges.

Wrongful death statutes vary from state to state. Today about 25 states allow fetuses to recover for wrongful death, even when stillborn. Most of these states[13] require that the fetus be viable at the time of injury.

Criminal Law

Some states[14] have passed laws making the destruction of the fetus punishable under criminal law; and the punishments are similar to those doled out for murder.[15] Yet, even in criminal law there are inconsistencies with regard to the status of the fetus: For in *State v Dickinson* the court found that a fetus that is never born is not a life legally entitled to protection; it must be born alive to be the victim of a homicide.[16]

According to the Model Penal Code, the definition of "homicide" is "causing the death of another human being," while the definition of "human being" is "a person who has been born and is alive."[17] If these definitions were adopted by all states, the fetus would not be protected by laws applying to persons unless it was subsequently born alive. However, states are enpowered to create their own definitions of these terms and to apply them to whomever they see fit. This has allowed for, and fostered, confusion and discord in awarding fetal protection under criminal law.

Constitutional Law

Courts have differed with regard to whether the fetus is entitled to protection as guaranteed to "persons" by the Constitution. The status of the fetus varies from state to state. In *McGarvey v Magee*, the court held that there was no indication that the framers of the Constitution intended to protect "fetal life" when drafting the Constitution.[18] Another case decided in the same year, *Byrn v New York*, found that children *in utero* need not be recognized as legal persons or entities entitled, under the state and federal constitutions, to a right to life.[19] However in the same year, 1972, (one year before the *Roe v Wade* decision was handed down) a court in Indiana found that " . . . a state interest in what is, at the very least, from the moment of conception a living being and potential human life, is both valid and compelling."[20]

1973

Until the early 1970's, the court system had managed to avoid direct confrontation of the issues of fetal personhood in tort law, criminal law, and constitutional law. In lower courts a trend toward the denial of rights to an unviable fetus seemed to exist, while they seemed generally willing to grant protection to the viable fetus.

However, in 1973 the Supreme Court in *Roe v Wade* held that a state could not adopt a concept of the fetus that could inhibit a woman's right to obtain an abortion. Again, the fetus was defined as not only a part of its mother, but also as secondary. In other words, a state could not find that conception, for example, was the point at which life began, and therefore the point at which personhood was granted to the fetus, because that could restrict a woman's ability to procure an abortion. *Roe* revolutionized the way in which a fetus was perceived in the law, especially in relation to the woman who carried it and the guarantees of her constitutional rights. Roe made it clear that a woman's rights to privacy and to bodily integrity could not be subjugated to those of an unviable fetus in any circumstance; nor did those rights automatically secondary once a fetus becomes viable.

Summary

The legal precedents that enable the fetus to apply for protection under inheritance law, tort law, criminal law, and constitutional law were intended to guard the fetus and, more importantly, the woman carrying it from harm by third persons. Women and their fetuses were seen as having sympathetic interests. Legal protection and recognition for the fetus was not intended to foster litigiousness between women and fetuses, but rather to protect pregnant women from " . . . having their pregnancies involuntarily and violently terminated by third parties."[21]

While it is true that the majority of women who are prosecuted for drug use during pregnancy are tried and/or convicted after they give birth (i.e. once the fetus is no longer a fetus), the drugs were passed from mother to child while it was still a fetus in utero. Yet, the *fetus* is not entitled to protection under drug trafficking or child abuse statutes.

This history will help to clarify the inadequacies in the policy of prosecuting women who used drugs during pregnancy. To clarify: First, there is a fetus, an entity that is not entitled to legal protection, who is being exposed to drugs while in utero. No laws on any books indicate that it is explicity illegal to pass drugs from mother to fetus. (Of course, that does not illigitimate the tragedy of it.) Then, after roughly ine months, there is anewborn, who is not only suddenly entitled to legal protection, but is also no longer being exposed to drugs. (It is now sustainig itself outside its mother.) Therefore, there technically is no crime beig committed. In the

same way that this analysis abandons tthe fetus to a
cruel legal limbo, the criminal prosecution of women
who use drugs during pregnancy condemns pregnant
addicts to a similar fate with limited access to pre-natal
care and to treatment. In order to avoid these catch-22's,
a more comprehensive social policy must be adopted.
Still, the following exploration will further elucidate the
inanity of the current trend toward prosecution.

THE RIGHTS OF THE WOMAN

An individual's right to control her own body has a
longstanding legal tradition. The very basic biological
fact that a fetus is, for nine months, a part of a woman's
body, means that any practice which places a fetus ahead
of its mother threatens a woman's constitutionally
protected rights to privacy and bodily integrity. Efforts to
prosecute women who use drugs during pregnancy are
closely linked to efforts to rob women of their rights to
control their reproductive freedom by an ideology that
denies women's autonomy and instead places control
over reproduction in the hands of the state. For the only
right that must be recognized to see that prosecuting
women for using drugs during pregnancy is not only
not sound as a legal policy but also as a social policy is a
woman's right to privacy. Legal privacy, much like the
legal status of the fetus, is socially and politically
defined. "The limits of the right of privacy are found by
examining societal values and determining which
private activities are traditionally sanctioned and which
proscribed."[22]

The rights of privacy have been protected by the
courts since the early 1800s. Over the past 150 years, the
courts have examined and re-examined privacy; old

limits were extended and new limits set. These re-
evaluations are constantly taking place as both the state
and individuals find new battlegrounds on which to
clash.

The court's 1965 opinion in *Griswold v
Connecticut*[23] presents the most comprehensive
assessment of privacy precedents. (Is it a coincidence that
this case, too, is about reproductive freedom?)
According to Justice Douglas, " . . . [s]pecific guarantees
in the Bill of Rights have penumbras . . . various
guarantees [that] create zones of privacy."[24] He listed the
First, Third, Fourth, Fifth and Ninth Amendments as
incorporating a constitutionally protected right to
privacy that was broad enough to encompass
childbearing decisions such as whether to use
contraception. In this case and in *Roe v Wade*,[25] which
legalized abortion, the justices of the Supreme Court
had a long list of privacy precedents on which to fall
back.

As early as 1891, the Supreme Court recognized the
right of bodily autonomy: "No right is more sacred, or is
more carefully guarded . . . than the right of every
individual to the possession and control of his [sic] own
person, free from all restraint or interference by others,
unless by clear and unquestionable authority of law."[26]
In *Olmstead v United States*, Justice Brandeis offered a
dissenting opinion: "The makers of our
constitution . . . conferred, as against the government,
the right to be left alone. . . . "[27]

Compelling State Interest

With privacy recognized as a fundamental right of
persons that is protected by the Constitution, states
intending to pass laws that could infringe upon the right

to privacy were required to show that the law was
necessary, narrowly drawn, and served to protect a
previously recognized compelling state interest.[28]   The
constitutional guarantee in the Fourteenth Amendment
of due process requires courts to consider how intrusive
a state's attempt to regulate a certain behavior is when
determining whether or not that regulation violates any
constitutional right, including the right to privacy. The
courts are required to attempt to create a balance when
two constitutionally protected rights conflict. For
example, in *Griswold*, the Supreme Court found that
attempting to regulate a couple's use of birth control
would be too intrusive to justify. Consider how
intrusive state regulation of a woman's behavior during
pregnancy would be: the state would have to monitor
what a woman ate and drank and smoked, when and if
and with whom she had sex, her physical activity, and
her work habits.

In *Roe*, the Supreme Court acknowledged that a state
interest in the life of the fetus exists, and that it becomes
compelling at the beginning of the third trimester (or
sixth month) of pregnancy. The state interest in the fetus
prior to six months gestation can not be given priority
over a woman's right to procure an abortion under any
circumstances as long as the procedure is performed in
accordance with state medical regulations. Even in the
third trimester, during which the state interest can be
sufficient enough to restrict abortion, a woman is still
entitled to an abortion if it can save her life.[29] Even in
the final trimester of pregnancy, when the fetus is the
most viable, the woman's rights still outweigh those of
the fetus. In addition, *Roe* establishes that a fetus is not
a person entitled to protection under the law. The
woman or mother, on the other hand, is. When women
are prosecuted in a way that potentially criminalizes
their behavior during pregnancy, whether it be

smoking, drinking, having sex, or using controlled substances because of its effect on fetuses, the rights of women are subjugated to the rights of an unborn entitly that has never been entitled to full legal protection.

Putting the fetus before the woman in this way not only flies in the face of legal precedents but also has many dangerous repercussions: The restriction of abortion is just one possible consequence of the prosecution of women who use drugs during pregnancy because it prioritzes the rights of the fetus to be born drug-free over the rights of the woman to make decisions about her own body. It could also undermine society's commitment to making health care and drug treatment available to pregnant women. Chapter 2 will discuss the ways in which many of the cases brought against pregnant drug addicts or users charge women with crimes that are usually committed against persons, not fetuses. For example, charging a woman with delivering drugs to a minor because her baby tested positive for cocaine at birth establishes that the state perceives of the fetus as a minor, a child, entitled to protection. If these cases are successful and fetuses are considered "minors" who must fall under the protective arm of the law and the Constitution, then abortion, in the first and second trimesters as well as the third, can be construed as murder. And women could be considered wards of the state during their pregnanies.

Privacy and Parents

Women should also be protected from prosecution for their behavior during pregnancy by virtue of their status as parents. The rights of parents in deciding when, if, and how to raise children (f we must consider fetuses as children) are protected by privacy doctrines. In the

1920s the Supreme Court recognized the Fourteenth Amendment protection of certain "liberties," which included the right of people to marry and to have children and to decide how those children should be educated.[30]   *Meyer v Nebraska* was the first case to recognize the rights of parents to make medical decisions for their children without state interference. Many cases have shown that "[t]he protection against state intrusion afforded by the constitution is especially strong where issues of childbearing are involved."[31]   In *Carey v Population Services International*, the Supreme Court found that, "the Constitution protects individual decisions in matters of childbearing from unjustified intrusion by the state." One of the conclusions of this case was that the pregnant woman ought to be the one to make decisions regarding the care of her fetus.[32]

Privacy and Medicine

This freedom from government intrusion has been referred to as a right to "personal privacy and dignity," "personal security," and "bodily security and personal privacy."[33] The right to bodily integrity is guaranteed by the equal protection clause of the Constitution as well as by the substantive due process clause. Some cases have resulted in rulings that establish that these guarantees are sufficient to preclude a state from forcing a person, against her/his will, to submit to medical treatment or to follow medical advice.[34]

In no state is it a crime for a patient to disobey a doctor's orders. As early as 1914 in *Schloendorff v Society of New York Hospitals*, the court ruled that "medical treatment given without consent constitutes assault." A disregard for patients' refusal of medical treatment can be construed as assault and/or battery depending on the state.[35]

In addition, forcing a patient to undergo medical treatment to which she/he objects, whether it be for religious reasons or otherwise, is now considered to be unacceptable medical procedure in light of the *Schloendorff* decision. In 1964, the Court forced two Jehovah's Witnesses to have blood transfusions, which were considered to be necessary for the preservation of their lives, against their wishes. Today, it is understood that these decisions do not reflect the "current emphasis on respect for individual self-determination and bodily integrity in medical decision-making."[36]

In two cases the Court has found that the state cannot force a person to undergo medical treatment even to obtain criminal evidence. In one case it was necessary to pump a criminal suspect's stomach in order to obtain the evidence needed for a conviction; in the other, a suspect refused to undergo an operation to have a bullet removed and the court upheld his right of bodily integrity.[37] This right also extends to mental patients committed against their will. Even when considering the rights of individuals over whom the state usually exercises a great deal of control, like criminal suspects and mental patients, the courts have been unwilling to infringe upon these rights. Yet, somehow post-partum women are being drug tested without consent when they are merely *suspected* of having used drugs during pregnancy.[38]

In addition to protecting the rights of individuals to refuse medical treatment and to disobey a doctor's request for treatment, the courts have been unwilling to require a parent to put her/himself at medical risk to save the life of her/his child. Traditionally, the American legal system has not imposed physical burdens on one individual for the sake of another.[39] For example, the Court cannot require a parent to donate an organ or give blood to her/his child. In *Stallman v Youngquist* the Court stated, "A legal right to guarantee the mental and physical health of another has never before been recognized in law."[40]   An individual has a right to guard her/his bodily integrity, which overrides any compelling moral obligation to another individual. Again, why should women who are already suffering from addiciton be held responsible for the health of their fetuses?

The only cases in which the Court has found that medical treatment can be imposed by the state are in situations where the treatment affords a protection to the rest of society: in *Jacobsen v Massachusetts* the Court found that the state could force people to submit to vaccinations so as not to endanger the rest of society. The court explained that privacy, like all constitutionally protected rights, is limited. "Liberty secured by the Constitution of the United States does not impart an absolute right in each person to be at all times or in all circumstances wholly free from restraint. . . . "[41] The safety of society at large has been recognized as a compelling state interest, and as such is an acceptable reason for restricting an individual's right to privacy.

The *Stallman* decision appears sufficient to establish a woman's right to determine the course of her medical treatment, even if she should opt not to undergo treatment, including drug rehabilitation or detox, that could benefit her fetus. A pregnant women's rights should not be different than the rights of other individuals in this regard; the states' interest in protecting an individual fetus is not the same as the state's interest in protecting a large group of citizens from the repercussions of one person's actions, or even as guarding the rights of a single pregnant woman. Any situation in which a woman refuses to subject herself to situation in which a woman refuses to subject herself to treatment solely for the benefit of her fetus should be viewed through the *Stallman* lens rather than through the *Jacobsen* lens; one fetus does not constitute "society."

A NEW TREND:
THE WOMAN VERSUS THE FETUS

However, over the past ten years a new trend has emerged; the recognition of fetal rights is now being used to impinge upon the rights of pregnant women. The state has attempted to mediate between women and fetuses by consciously placing itself in the guardianship role. "The authority of courts to appoint representatives to protect fetal interests is now firmly established. Courts of general equitable jurisdiction are imbued with ample power to appoint guardians . . . for unborn children in a variety of circumstances."[42] The courts have begun to recognize the legal rights of the fetus "to *begin* life with a sound mind and body."[43]

In the early 1980s, doctors began looking to the courts in order to force women to undergo treatment against their will to benefit the fetus. In these instances doctors have claimed that they have an obligation, shared by the state, to protect the interests of the fetus. This is why medical professionals have turned to the court for permission to violate a patients right to bodily integrity; they do not want to accept responsibility for these kinds of invasions which have been construed as illegal and unconstitutional in the past. This trend encompasses many issues of reproductive freedom from court-ordered caesarian sections to an effort to restrict access to abortion. This will be further discussed in Chapter 2.

Roe v Wade

It is important to examine the history of *Roe v Wade* here because its evolution and its demise are symptomatic of the sentiment that has made prosecution on the basis of behavior during pregnancy a very real threat.

Privacy, Bodily Integrity and the Fetus

As explained above, in order for a state to infringe upon an individual's right to bodily autonomy and privacy it must show a compelling, *previously recognized,* state interest. (For example, the protection of society in the vaccination case is a valid state interest.) Therefore the question of whether a state can intervene on behalf of a fetus in a woman's pregnancy can only be answered by considering the state's *previously recognized* interest in the fetus.

In the brief for the appellant in *Roe v Wade*, which dealt directly with Texas statutes, the lawyers explained that if the state has an interest in protecting the fetus as a motivation for illegalizing abortion, then other statutes should protect that fetal life, too. Did they? No. In Texas, in 1972, a woman was not considered an accomplice in an abortion, self-abortion was not considered a crime, nor was travelling to another state to obtain an abortion. Fetuses were not protected by homicide laws in Texas. And no formalities of death were reported for fetuses fewer than five months old. "[T]he state has no *traditional* interest in protection of the fetus. If an interest exists, it must be relatively recent in its discovery."[44]

In contrast, the state has consistently and repeatedly asserted a compelling interest in protecting children. Under the doctrine of *parens patriae*, the state's right to use its police powers to provide for the protection and care of children is well established. It "enable[s] state[s] to provide for the welfare of minors and incompetents who would otherwise be miscared for."[45]   The policy implications of this are clear: every state has enacted and enforced, with the support of the federal government, child abuse and neglect laws which give the state the right to infringe upon the relationship of the parent and her/his child if it is deemed to be in the best interest of the child.   Remember that the fetus does not become a child until *after* it is born.

To this end, the courts have often become involved in medical situations where parents, for whatever reason, refuse to give their consent for medical treatment for their children. The courts tend to override the decision of the parents; but, here, too, there is room for variation as courts respect more and more the decisions of competent adults.[46]   Nevertheless, the state's interest in protecting children is "traditional" as well as "compelling" and "justified."

Regardless of whether the state interest in the fetus was "traditional" or "recent in its discovery," *Roe* has now established a compelling state interest in protecting the life of the fetus that emerges at viability. The 1973 Supreme Court reached the conclusion that a fetus became viable, for the purposes of establishing a state interest, at the end of the sixth month of pregnancy, also known as the beginning of the third trimester. Thus, fetal rights are now recognized and protected in some capacity, albeit inconsistently, by almost every state.

The Constitutional Balancing Act:

In any contest between two constitutionally protected rights, the Supreme Court is required to balance one against the other in an effort to preserve, as much as possible, the sanctity of each. So, since the Court decided to recognize that the right of a woman to control her own body entitled her to access to abortion, the central issue in *Roe v Wade* was how to balance the legal rights of the fetus examined above with the rights of a woman to bodily integrity and privacy. The Fourteenth Amendment to the Constitution protects individuals' freedom from unwarranted bodily restraint. A majority of states find a compelling interest in protecting the rights of the fetus, and many courts have been willing to validate that interest when it is beneficial to already born persons. Abortion in the context of maternal-fetal conflict, raises a new set of questions because it sets the interests of the fetus and the interests of the woman in opposition to one another.

The Supreme Court in *Roe* did not really address the issue of the legal standing of the fetus. Rather, it established "viability," a medically determined distinction, as the fulcrum of the scale that balances a woman's constitutional right to privacy against the state's right to intervene on behalf of the fetus. *Roe* ensured that women would be able to procure abortions in the first trimester of pregnancy on demand, during the second trimester with increased regulation by the state, and in the third trimester only when her life was endangered. Blackmun's opinion found that the state's interest in protecting fetal life became compelling enough to prevent women from making major life decisions about whether or not to bear children only after viability.[47] From 1973, when *Roe* was decided, until 1989, women enjoyed a constitutionally protected right to privacy that was broad enough to encompass the decision to have an abortion. Through 1989 the Supreme Court continued to maintain that any state interest in protecting the potential life of the fetus must be subject to the state concerns for the health and safety of the woman.[48]~

The *Roe* triumph catalyzed anti-abortion forces in this country to work for a repeal of *Roe* and the recriminalization of abortion as well as to gain legal recognition for the fetus as a person entitled to protection under the law.

In 1989, they got their opportunity. The Supreme Court heard *Webster v Reproductive Health Services* which challenged, among other efforts to restrict access to abortion, the Missouri state legislature's finding that life begins at conception. The Supreme Court, in a very different political setting than 1973, upheld Missouri's right to define life as beginning at conception. This decision sent the fight for control over women's bodies back to the state legislatures. Women still had a constitutional right to privacy that could enable them to legally procure an abortion, but the Supreme Court was willing to find the state's interest in protecting fetal life to be more compelling than it did in 1973. States were suddenly encouraged to adopt definitions and ideas about life and personhood that could grant the fetus full protection of its rights to life and liberty under state statutes.

While *Roe* recognized the rights of the fetus as compelling at viability, *Webster* established that the Supreme Court was willing to defend the state's interest in protecting the potentiality of life throughout pregnancy.[49] Whether state efforts to restrict abortion are motivated by a concern for the protection of the fetus or are part of a larger effort to restrict the rights of women remains to be seen.

The most recent focus of the struggle over the rights of the fetus has shifted toward pregnant women who choose to carry to term and away from women who chose to abort. In the wake of *Webster*, states have begun to champion the rights of fetuses not just against third parties, nor against women who want to terminate their unwanted pregnancies, but over the rights of pregnant women who have chosen to give birth. "*Webster* can be interpreted as enabling states to promulgate extensive interventions in order to protect the health of fetus, as long as the pregnant woman evidences an intent to continue her pregnancy."[50]

In the interim between *Roe* and *Webster* , states sought to infringe upon a woman's rights to privacy and bodily integrity by obtaining judicial sponsorship of forced medical procedures, such as Caesarian sections, to protect the life of the fetus. Since *Webster,* the battle has intensified: an examination of the recent cases brought by states prosecuting women for their behavior during pregnancy and a discussion of the current debate over the need for these criminal prosecutions can shed some light on the motivations of the state and why states have chosen to pursue fetal protection through the prosecution of women.

However, to deliver healthy babies pregnant women must have access to pre-natal healthcare and drug treatment. Despite the fact that there is in an inadequate supply of these resources, the courts have begun to hold women solely responsible when their children are born with defects that can be linked to their behavior during pregnancy. Viewing women and fetuses as separate entities with distinct interests is dangerous because it forces fetuses to compete against their mothers for protection under the law, rather than helping women and fetuses to receive better care. Pitting women and their fetuses against one another also jeopardizes the rights of women to privacy and bodily integrity.

NOTES

[1] Dawn E. Johnsen, "The Creation of Fetal Rights: Conflicts With Women's Constitutional Rights to Liberty, Privacy and Equal Protection,"*Yale Law Journal* 95 (1986): 599.

[2] 410 U. S. 113, at 162 (1973).

[3] Ibid, at 161.

[4] Johnsen, 614.

[5] Johnsen, 603.

[6] Westfall, "Beyond Abortion: the Potential Reach of the Human Life Amendment," *Defining Human Life: Medical, Legal, and Ethical Implications*, eds. Marjery Shaw and A. Edward Doudera (AUPHA Press, 1983)187.

[7] Cowles v Cowles 56 Conn. 240 (1887); Medlock v Brown 163 Ga. 520 (1927); McLain v Howald 120 Mich. 271 (1899); Christian v Carter 193 N. C. 537 (1927).

[8] 138 Mass. 14 (1884).

[9] Viability, as a distinct point, is medically determined. Therefore, it is a movable reference point. As medical technology advances, the point at which the fetus can be sustained outside its mother grows increasingly early in pregnancy. Today, medical technology can successfully sustain a 20-21-week-old fetus.

[10] 65 F. Supp. 138 (1946).

[11] 38 N.W. 2d 838 (1949).

[12] Cheryl E. Amana, "Ethical and Legal Considerations of Maternal-Fetal Conflict in the Context of Substance Abuse" (Master's Essay, Columbia University, School of Law, 1990), 10.

[13] Rhode Island and Georgia allow actions for wrongful death prior to viability.

[14] California, Illinois, Iowa, Michigan, Mississippi, New Hampshire, Oklahoma, Utah, Washington, and Wisconsin include destruction of the fetus in their criminal codes.

[15] Johnsen, 604.

[16] 275 N.E. 2d 599 (1971).

[17] R. Meyers, "Abuse and Neglect of the Unborn," *Duquesne Law Review* 23 (1984): 12-13.

[18] 340 F. Supp. 751 (1972).

[19] 31 N.Y. 2d 194 (1972).

[20] Cheany v State 285 N.E. 2d 265, at 270 (1972).

[21] Johnsen, 603.

[22] Meyers, 56.

[23] 381 U.S. 484 (1964). Estelle Griswold, the Executive Director of Connecticut Planned Parenthood was tried and convicted for operating a birth control clinic in Connecticut. She successfully appealed her case. Planned Parenthood had been trying to change Connecticut law banning the dissemination of birth control information and its distribution for years.

[24] 381 U.S. 484, at 596 (1964).

[25] 410 U. S. 113 (1973).

[26] Union Pacific Railroad v Botsford 141 U.S. 250, at 251 (1891).

[27] 277 U. S. 438 (1927).

[28] Molly McNulty, "Pregnancy Police: The Health Policy and Legal Implications of Punishing Pregnant Women for Harm to their Fetuses," *New York University Review of Law and Social Change*, 16 (1987-1988): 315. See Skinner 316 U.S. 535, at 540-1 (1942) and Akron 462 U.S. 416, at 427 (1983).

[29] During the first trimester or up to approximately 12 weeks of pregnancy the rights of the woman are strongest. The state may not interfere in a woman's decision to abort. During the second trimester, from twelve weeks to roughly twenty-four weeks, the state may regulate abortion *only* to protect the health of the woman. Here the "compelling state interest" is the women's health. After twenty-four weeks (which is approximately when a fetus was considered to be viable in 1973) the state's compelling interest becomes the protection of the fetus and this interest overrides the rights of the women; the state may prohibit abortion entirely, except when the women's life is endangered.

[30] See Meyer v Nebraska 262 U.S. 390 (1923) and Pierce v Society of Sisters 268 U.S. 510 (1925).

[31] Johnsen, 617. See Griswold v Connecticut 381 U.S. 479 (contraception); Loving v Virginia 388 U.S. 1 (marriage); Eisenstadt v Baird 405 U.S. 438 (contraception for unmarried persons); Roe v Wade 410 U.S. 113 (abortion).

[32] 431 U.S. 678, at 685 (1977).

[33] Johnsen, 615.

[34] See In Re Quinlan 355 A.2d 647; In Re Conroy 486 A.2d 1209; and Saikewicz 370 N.E. 2d 417.

35 V. Kolder et al., "Court Ordered Obstetrical Interventions," *New England Journal of Medicine* (7 May 1987), 1195.

36 Ibid.

37 See Rochin v California and Winston v Lee.

38 The majority of women who are drug tested are suspected of drug use/abuse during pregnancy on the basis of one or more of the following conditions: premature birth, low birth weight, or lack of prenatal care. These conditions are often related to socio-econimic class and race. For a moe in depth discussion of these issues, see Chapter 2.

39 Janet Gallagher, "The Fetus and the Law," *Ms.*, September 1984, 66.

40 Stallman v. Youngquist, 531 N.E. 2d 355, at 359. (Ill. 1988).

41 197 U.S. 11 (1904).

42 see Taft v Taft 446 N.E. 2d 395 (1983). This practice follows from English common law and is well established in American legal history.

43 Stallman v Youngquist 531 N.E. 2d 355, at 358. (Ill. 1988).

44 Brief for Appellant in Roe v Wade, 121.

45 Amana, 11-12.

46 Gallagher, 64.

47 In Roe viability was considered to be the point at which the fetus could exist on its own, outside the mother. In 1973 twenty-four weeks was the earliest point at which this could happen. Medical advances have now pushed that point back to somewhere between twenty and twenty-one weeks.

48   Thornburgh v American College of Obstetricians and Gynecologists 106 S. Ct. 2169 (1986).

49   Webster v Reproductive Health Services 109 S.Ct. 3040, at 3055-56 (1989).

50   Amana, 3-4.

II

The Emergence of Fetal Rights into the Mainstream

From 1973 until the early 1980s women enjoyed the right to control their reproductive lives; *Roe v Wade* made that possible when it legalized abortion. This chapter examines the emergence of fetal rights into the mainstream that began in the early 1980s.

Some early efforts to champion the rights of the unborn resulted in an increase in medical procedures performed on pregnant women against their will. As advancements in the fields of neonatology and perinatology allowed doctors greater access to information about the development of the fetus; the point of viability was pushed back. Sonograms, which enabled doctors and mothers to actually see the fetus in utero became common practice. As the fetus developed into a accessible, treatable patient, whose interests could be addressed separately from the mother's, doctors became more willing to see the fetus as a patient in its own right. [1]

These developments led some doctors to challenge women's rights to make their own medical decisions during pregnancy. Doctors began seeking court orders to perform Caesarian sections on pregnant women in their care when the doctor believed that a woman's choice in

29

accepting or refusing medical care did not place the health of the fetus above her own well-being. These doctors can be seen as attempting to protect their patients, fetuses, who were unable to speak for themselves. However, the effect of this intervention was to prioritize the safety of the fetus, and devalue the woman's right to bodily integrity.

By the mid-1980s some county law enforcement officials, confronted with an increase in babies born addicted to drugs, began to criminally prosecute women for their behavior during pregnancy that resulted in harm to their fetuses. Here the courts were reluctant at first get involved and many cases were dismissed. But, within a few years, due to rising infant mortality and increasing female autonomy, as evidenced by increased female workforce participation and abortion rates, the courts were willing to punish women who had elected to carry to term and then not protected themselves and their fetuses from harm. Women who gave birth to unhealthy fetuses were investigated and brought before the criminal justice system where they were required to defend their actions.

This chapter will examine the emergence of forced Caesarian sections in the early 1980s. It will also follow the development of the crusade to prosecute drug-using mothers. At first states found that the courts were unwilling to back them up. However, as prosecutors refined and further defined the crimes of these women, the court seemed ready to put these women behind bars.

The criminal prosecution of women who use drugs during pregnancy may well have been conceived of as a way to eliminate, or at least reduce, drug use among pregnant women, thus reducing the number of babies born disadvantaged by pre-natal drug exposure. However, it has not done that yet, nor does it seem likely that it will. The underlying causes of these problems, as stated above, are more deeply rooted in society than drug use by these women; they include poverty, a lack of pre-natal health care, and inadequate drug treatment options (especially for pregnant women).

In addition, criminal prosecution of drug-using pregnant women amounts to the criminalization of drug addiction which is considered, both medically and legally, to be a disease and *not* a crime. Women who use drugs and become pregnant are not going to come forward for either pre-natal care or drug treatment at the risk of being prosecuted. Therefore, if the prosecution of these women becomes the norm rather than the unacceptable deviation women's needs for care might never be addressed as the real problem.

If prosecutors are concerned with eliminating drug use among pregnant women in order to protect fetuses, they should refocus their energies; perhaps they could put pressure on local, state, and federal politicians to appropriate funds to alleviate the underlying crises. However, if they are interested in restricting women's rights to control their own bodies and make childbearing decisions for themselves they are pursuing a most effective method.

Issues of race and class must be discussed for even though drug use during pregnancy cuts across racial and socio-economic lines, the majority of the women who are a) caught and b) prosecuted are poorer women of color. This provides evidence that these efforts in the name of "fetal rights" are really a concerted attempt to restrict the control women ought to legally have over their bodies. The fight for "fetal rights" can be seen as a state sponsored effort to appear to be addressing the larger social issues of poverty and inadequate health care and drug treatment. As there are two patients, there are two victims of drug use among pregnant women: the fetus and the woman. The methods discussed below prioritize the fetus and devalue the woman. This is not the way to solve the problem. The individual cases discussed below are enough to establish legal precedents that could have an impact on women all across the country for years to come.

THE DOCTORS AND THE COURTS: FORCED MEDICAL PROCEDURES

A 1987 article in the *New England Journal of Medicine* reported that health care institutions in eighteen states were aware of thirty-six attempts to override maternal refusals of medical treatment between 1982 and 1987.[2] These efforts included attempts to perform Caesarian sections and intra-uterine transfusions, as well as to obtain permission to detain a pregnant woman in the hospital against her will. The overwhelming majority of interventions were approved by the judges who presided over the proceedings.

Three hospital detentions were sought by doctors in two states (three total): Colorado and Illinois. One was granted in each state. Only one court order for a doctor to perform an intra-uterine transfusion on a woman against her will was granted. Fifteen court orders were sought for unwanted Caesarian sections between 1982 and 1987. Of the eleven states involved, all but one gave the doctor permission to proceed without the consent of the women. Colorado, Hawaii, Illinois, Minnesota, Michigan, Ohio, Tennessee, South Carolina, Tennessee, and Texas all allowed the women to be discounted in the medical decision making process. Maine was the only state of the eleven to find on behalf of the woman.

Despite the fact that not one of the women who had refused the medical treatment recommended by her doctor was ever declared incompetent through these proceedings, eighty-six percent of the court orders sought were obtained. In one Colorado case, reported in the *American Journal of Obstetrics and Gynecology*, the doctors called in a psychiatrist while a woman was in labor to have her declared incompetent when she refused to consent to a C-section. Although the psychologist declared her to be competent, the court order was sought and eventually granted by a juvenile court.[3] Eighty-eight percent of the court orders were obtained within six-hours: Clearly, neither the doctors nor the courts had any doubt as to whether or not it was legitimate to override a woman's refusal of medical care in order to protect her fetus.

The interventions reported in this survey targeted the disempowered members of our society: women, but specifically women who are on public assistance, women who are single, women who do not speak English as their primary language. Eighty-one percent of these cases involved African-American, Hispanic, or Asian women. Forty-four percent of them were single. Twenty-four percent were not entirely familiar with English. One hundred percent of these women were treated either in a teaching hospital or in a clinic and all of them were on public assistance of some kind.[4]

Chances are good that many, if not all, of these women did not have the support systems necessary to contest these invasions of their privacy; being patients on public aid and in public facilities certainly does not entitle them to individualized care Those women who had difficulty with the English language may have been unable to fully understand their options and/or the medical procedures that were being forced upon them. The single women may already have had children that they needed to care for and were unable to devote the time for surgery and recuperation without disadvantaging these already existing children.

It is not necessary to speculate further on the details of these women's lives. Their common denominator is that they were all violated in a manner that would be unacceptable to men and even to non-pregnant women. Finally, most of them were entirely without the means to defend themselves legally.

However not all cases involve women of color and women on public assistance. Two specific examples can provide an illustration of the extent to which the rights of the fetus can be championed over the rights, and even the dignity, of the woman. In June, 1987 Angela Carder, a twenty-eight-year-old, middle-class, white woman was diagnosed with lung cancer. She was 26 weeks pregnant. Despite the fact that her doctors advised her that a Caesarian section could be fatal for Angela, the hospital, George Washington University Hospital, sought a court order for a C-section. Angela refused to consent to the procedure. Her doctors and her family supported her in her decision not to have the surgery. The trial court in the District of Columbia ordered the Caesarian section. The baby was delivered ten weeks premature, and died almost immediately. Angela Carder died two days later. Perhaps the hospital was hoping to preserve some life; a doctor predicted that the fetus was sufficiently viable to survive the C-section, but the effects of his misjudgement were to not only terminate Angela's pregnancy against her will, but also to deprive her of the remainder of her privacy, autonomy and, ultimately, her life.

Her family decided to appeal the case despite Angela's death. The Court of Appeals agreed to hear the case because it considered the situation to be "capable of happening again yet, evading review."[5] The Court of Appeals vacated the trial court's decision in April 1990. The opinion strongly supported the rights of a woman to control her own medical care: "We hold that in virtually all cases the question of what is to be done is to be decided by the patient—the pregnant woman—on behalf of herself and the fetus . . . a fetus can not have rights in this respect superior to those of a person who has already been born."[6]

In another example of court ordered medical intervention, the Georgia Supreme Court recognized a viable fetus as being entitled to the protection of the state's Juvenile Court Code. In this case, *Jefferson v Griffin Spalding County Hospital Authority* [7], a Georgia woman with a placenta previa, a condition that means that she would be unable to give birth vaginally without her placenta detaching from the uterine wall, was forced to undergo a Caesarian section against her religious belief that precluded surgery as well as blood transfusions. (This condition is dangerous for the woman as well; she could bleed to death if her placenta detaches from the uterine wall. But she should still be entitled to choose to take this risk.) In this case, the Court declared that the fetus was capable of sustaining life outside its mother (i.e. it was viable) and as a result, was being deprived of "proper care and sustenance." In a court of law, this was a defeat for the plaintiff; however, this story has a happy ending. Ms. Jefferson's placenta shifted before the surgery was performed and a healthy baby was delivered vaginally.

According to the *American Journal of Obstetrics and Gynecology*, this was a precedent-setting case. Its effect was to inform doctors that "their duties to the fetus as a 'patient' might authorize surgery on a pregnant woman even though she refused to consent."[8] These two cases illustrate how health care professionals and the judicial systems are capable of working together in order to save the life of a fetus and deprive women of their traditionally protected rights to bodily integrity; they also illustrate how both doctors and judges can be wrong in attempting to protect fetuses by setting up a competition between a mother and her fetus.

Court ordered medical procedures on pregnant women have been condemned in many forums. Publications as varied as *U.S. News and World Report, Glamour, Ms., The Nation,* and *The New England Journal of Medicine* have run articles over the past decade decrying the invasion of pregnant women's bodies. In addition, the American College of Obstetricians and Gynecologists and the American Medical Association both issued statements opposing court ordered medical treatment, like Caesarian sections. According to the American Public Health Association, "Rather than protecting the health of women and children, court-ordered C-sections erode the element of trust that permits a pregnant women to communicate to her physician—without fear of reprisal—all information relevant to her proper diagnosis and treatment."[9]

Civil liberties organizations including the American Civil Liberties Union (ACLU) have also come out against medical-judicial interventions such as these, calling them violations of otherwise constitutionally protected rights. To distill the arguments in favor of forced medical procedures: if a woman decides to carry her pregnancy to term, rather than have an abortion, she effectively forfeits her rights to control her own body.[10] If a woman does not see abortion as an option, because she can not afford it or can not obtain spousal or parental consent, then she is forced into relinquishing control over her pregnancy. These forced medical treatments demonstrate that pregnant women are treated differently than others with regard to the traditional doctor-patient relationship, and to the long-standing, judicially upheld right of patients to direct their own medical care. Many human rights advocates, as well as women's rights advocates, see this tendency among some doctors to use courts as the first phase of a campaign to reduce women to childbearing "vessels." These cases illustrate the attempts of a few medical professionals to gain control over the objections of the primary medical patient: the mother.

THE DISTRICT ATTORNEYS AND THE COURTS: CRIMINAL PROSECUTION OF WOMEN FOR THEIR BEHAVIOR DURING PREGNANCY

In the same way that some medical professionals have attempted to use their medical knowledge to protect fetuses, some local law enforcement officials are attempting to use their police powers to campaign for fetal rights. The result has been the emergence of the criminal prosecution of women who use drugs during pregnancy as a means of acting on the crisis of drug babies in hospitals around the country. Unfortunately for everyone involved, this method is questionable: Does it in fact protect fetuses, newborns and children from drug-using mothers? Or does it hurt them by separating them from their parents and placing them in the already over-extended child welfare system? Does it encourage women to stop using drugs and seek treatment? Or does it drive them further away from care and threaten to deprive them of their rights? These questions can be answered by examining the prosecutions that have taken place in the past few years.

By the beginning of 1990, there were at least thirty-five instances in which women were being criminally prosecuted for their conduct during pregnancy.[11] Most of these cases involve women with substance abuse problems whose newborns were exposed *in utero* to these chemicals. District Attorneys in states around the country have become involved in identifying these women and charging them with crimes ranging from disobeying doctors' orders, to criminal child abuse and neglect, to delivering illicit drugs to a minor. The methods of prosecution have varied from state to state as prosecutors met with failure in front of judges who were unwilling to include fetuses within the definition of "child" or "minor." As time passed and the rate of babies born exposed to drugs continued to increase, District Attorneys became increasingly meticulous in their approaches to these prosecutions.

Dr. Wendy Chavkin, at the Columbia University School of Public Health, explained that there are three basic approaches used to involve the law in forcing a "duty of care" upon pregnant women. In some instances, when drugs are detected in the mother's body (after the child is born), the case is reported to social service officials or law enforcement officials who then work to determine whether the child should be removed from the care and custody of its mother. Dr. Chavkin says that these types of cases are happening all over the country. Other efforts are aimed at pregnant women who enter the criminal justice system for other reasons, such as shoplifting or drug dealing. These women are punished more harshly than they would be if they were not pregnant and using drugs simultaneously. Thirdly, many jurisdictions have begun testing the urine of newborns who demonstrate signs of drug exposure not only to treat the infant, but also to determine if their mothers have been using drugs during pregnancy.[12]

A First Effort

The first time criminal law was involved in the maternal-fetal relationship was in 1985 in the case of Pamela Rae Stewart, a twenty-seven-year-old women from El Cajon, California. Nine months after she gave birth, Harry Elias, San Diego County Deputy District Attorney, charged Stewart with a misdemeanor: "willfully failing to provide necessary care for her child." A conviction for misdemeanor child neglect in El Cajon carries a punishment of up to $2,000 in fines and one year in jail.

The background in this case is important because it provides an illustration of the invasive methods employed by the police and the Child Protective Services to uncover evidence against Pamela Stewart. This case is also indicative of the condition of pre-natal health care in this country and the enthusiasm with which women are blamed for circumstances often beyond their control.

Like so many poor women in this country, Pamela Rae Stewart received little pre-natal care; the doctor who did examine her found that she had a placenta previa: This condition can lead to maternal hemorrhaging and fetal deprivation of oxygen. Stewart's doctor warned her against having sex and against using street drugs, and he also advised her to call the hospital immediately should she begin to bleed.

Her son, Thomas, was born with brain damage. He was released from the hospital five weeks later and placed in a foster home. Paul Zlotnik, the Medical

Director at the Neonatal Intensive Care Unit at
Grossmont Hospital, provided the impetus for the
criminal investigation of the Stewart case. He was not
Stewart's doctor. Zlotnik had ordered a toxicology
screening on Thomas when he was born; the results
revealed traces of amphetamines. The toxicology
performed on Stewart revealed the presence of
marijuana and amphetamines in her system. Despite
the fact that consent was not given for either of the tests,
Zlotnik reported the findings to the Child Protective
Services (CPS) which then began an investigation.

CPS then handed the case over to the Police
Department. Once Harry Elias became involved, he left
no stone unturned while searching for evidence to
convict Pamela Stewart. In conducting his investigation,
Elias also paid no attention to Stewart's constitutional
rights of privacy. The ACLU considers the way in which
Elias obtained Stewart's medical records to be a violation
of her constitutionally protected rights to privacy. He
used her doctor's medical reports as evidence in her
prosecution, which not only violated the confidentiality
of the doctor-patient relationship., but also violated
Stewart's right to non-disclosure of her medical records.

When Stewart was finally arrested and charged, Elias
relied on these medical reports, which were obtained in
apparent violation of Stewart's rights, and on the
testimony of her own husband, Thomas Monson. Dr.
Zlotnik informed Elias that Monson admitted that, in
his opinion, Stewart was negligent. Monson told Dr.
Zlotnik that Stewart had not taken her medicine as she
had been instructed, that *the two of them* had had
sexual intercourse, and that she had used street drugs,
all against the advice of her doctor. In Elias's mind this
added up to a violation of a 1925 California child
support statute.

The Municipal Court Judge E. MacAmos dismissed the case on February 26, 1987, before it had a chance to get to trial for this reason; he said the prosecution had used the wrong statute. The 1925 statute did provide for the protection of children "conceived but not yet born," however it was intended to protect *women* by requiring men to support their children.[13] In other words the statute was designed to punish fathers for abandoning mothers and children, even those children still *in utero*. (Recall Chapter 1 which discussed laws that were designed to protect fetuses conceived but not yet born from harm by third parties.) Judge MacAmos explained that the statute did criminalize the withholding of medical care from a child and that fetuses were indeed explicitly included in the definition of a "child" under this law, but he explained that it applied to women who were seeking financial support from their estranged husbands. His opinion continued, recommending that the state pass a law protecting the unborn from abuse by its mother.[14]

So, the judge was unwilling to punish Stewart for her behavior during her pregnancy under a misconstrued statute but, as his opinion indicates, he would not have dismissed the case if the law had provided for such a prosecution. (Legislative efforts to respond to such judicial appeals will be discussed later in this chapter.) In essence, Pamela Rae Stewart was prosecuted for disobeying her doctor's orders to the detriment of the health of her newborn child. As a first effort to force legal responsibility for the unborn upon women it was unsuccessful; but it did provide momentum and hope for success in the future. Health care professionals, social service workers, and law enforcement agents worked together; the effect was to bring Pamela Rae Stewart into the criminal justice system and charge her with a crime against her fetus.

These allegiances are dangerous because they blur the boundaries between public and private domains.

Once the prosecution of Pamela Rae Stewart had failed, jurisdictions around the country began to develop more creative strategies in an attempt to dictate what constitutes acceptable behavior during pregnancy. Prosecutors turned to criminal laws which prohibit delivering drugs to minors, assault with a deadly weapon (the umbilical cord?), or involuntary manslaughter. Some courts seized custody of fetuses *in utero* which enabled them to put women, arrested for some other, unrelated crime, in jail for the duration of their pregnancies to protect the interests of the fetus.

These efforts were largely inconsistent and unsuccessful, but they make clear that the goal of these prosecutions, to protect fetuses from exposure to drugs, could only be achieved at the expense of the freedom of these women. It is also possible to view these prosecutions as an attempt to define and impose a socially defined standard of behavior for pregnant women by encouraging states to monitor and then to judge a pregnant women's behavior.

Race and Class

Despite the fact that drug use during pregnancy crosses all socio-economic and racial boundaries, the majority of the women who have been prosecuted are minority women as well as women who are impoverished and dependent on public assistance. This is an important factor in analyzing the criminal prosecution of women who use drugs during pregnancy because these women are forced to use public facilities to receive care; they are unable to afford private care and the accompanying assurances of confidentiality.

The threat of criminal prosecution for drug use during pregnancy is even more dangerous to women who have few options. Even if a woman on public assistance wants to get into a drug rehabilitation program she is usually unable to do so; as mentioned above, most programs do not even accept pregnant women, and those that do have waiting lists of up to eighteen months. In many ways, "for a woman accused of pre-natal child abuse, the only option to avoid prosecution or imprisonment may be an abortion."[15] Women who rely on public assistance do not even have this option because abortions are not covered by medicaid. When a woman is dependant on public assistance, like so many of the women being prosecuted are, she can not rely on the doctor to protect her confidentiality. If a private doctor were to release information about a patient's drug use, a lawyer would be able to invalidate that evidence on the basis of a privacy violation.[16] Advocates of criminalization have realized that poor women, women who have no options, no treatment, no chance to terminate their pregnancies, and no resources to defend themselves, are more likely to have contact with public authorities and more likely to be drug tested (as a result of discriminatory screening procedures) and therefore more likely to be charged and then convicted.

The demographic characteristics of the women who have been prosecuted indicate that prosecutors are fully aware of the impact these conditions have on their chances of obtaining a conviction. In Pinellas County, Florida, for example, where drug use cuts across racial and socio-economic lines, African-American pregnant drug users are ten times as likely as white users to be reported to state agencies.[17] Dorothy E. Roberts, an associate professor of criminal law and civil liberties at Rutgers University who specializes in the reproductive rights of women of color, sees the prosecution of pregnant women drug users as a way to punish poor women for having babies. "This policy means that not only does our society tell poor inner-city women that we will not recognize your right to choose to have an abortion, we will not recognize your right to have a healthy pregnancy, but if you are a drug addict, we will punish you for having a baby."[18]She identifies this trend as part of a longstanding tradition of the devaluation of black motherhood: From forced breeding during slavery to forced sterilization, to the denial of custody rights, to the present campaign.[19]To wit, an ACLU memorandum on a survey of prosecutions brought against pregnant women disclosed that 80 percent were brought against women of color.[20] Dr. Ira Chasnoff of the National Association for Perinatal Addiction, Research and Education (NAPARE) attributes this disparity in prosecutions to widely held, discriminatory, ideas of "who a drug abuser is."

These issues again force a challenge of the stated goals of the prosecution of women who use drugs during pregnancy. Indeed, as Roberts asks, citing infant mortality rates, "If the government were truly concerned about the health of Black infants why hasn't there been a material commitment to ensuring that pregnant women in poor communities receive high quality pre-natal care?"[21]

Other Efforts

In 1988 the District Attorney for Butte County, California announced that county hospitals would begin testing all newborns suspected of being exposed to controlled substances *in utero*. According to this D.A., Michael Ramsey, a positive test result would lead to criminal prosecution of the mother for illegal drug use. In California, this is a misdemeanor that is punishable by mandatory drug treatment or ninety days in jail. Ramsey explained that his tactic constituted a creative use of the law by depending on the evidence obtained through drug testing of newborn to prove that a woman had used illegal drugs.[22] Ramsey was not the only D.A. to use "creative" techniques to prosecute drug-using pregnant women.

In Broward County, Florida, Tonia Hudson was arraigned for delivering drugs to a minor when her baby was born with cocaine it its body.

In North Carolina, in 1990, a prosecutor charged a woman with assault with a deadly weapon when her newborn's toxicology test was positive.

In February 1989, Melanie Green of Rockford, Illinois was arrested and charged with involuntary manslaughter and delivering drugs to a minor when her daughter died of oxygen deprivation two days after she was born and the baby's urine tested positive for cocaine. Melanie Green, an African-American woman, was the first woman in this country to be charged with manslaughter for the death of a child due to drug use during pregnancy. The prosecutor, Paul Logli, who is the Winnebago County State Attorney, asserted that Melanie's case was not "a pro-choice or a pro-life case. [It dealt] with a child who was born and lived two days."[23] Still, the Grand Jury refused to indict Melanie Green. After this case, the Illinois state legislature passed the Infant Neglect and Controlled Substances Act of 1989, making child abuse statutes applicable to newborns.

The women in these examples were prosecuted for their use of drugs during pregnancy which had a concrete *effect* on their newborns; these *effects* were the immediate motivating factors in instigating criminal proceedings against these women. The women involved were being judged on the basis of their actions; they had used controlled substances during pregnancy, and the use of these substances had damaged their newborn babies. At least these women had been allowed the autonomy to act throughout their pregnancies; the state wanted to become involved after a "crime" had been committed. In other cases the state acted to *prevent* the abuse of drugs during pregnancy. Consider these examples:

1981: A Louisiana juvenile court confines a woman to a hospital for the last two months of her pregnancy, claiming that it was taking jurisdiction of her fetus because a local welfare agency had reported that she was unable to care for it herself. A higher court later overturned this decision, but it was too late; the woman's confinement and her pregnancy were already over.[24]

1984: An Illinois judge sends a pregnant heroin user to drug rehabilitation after making her fetus a ward of the state because, according to the court, she was "abusing" it.[25]

1989: Brenda Vaughn is arrested and convicted in the District of Columbia of forging checks in the amount of roughly nine hundred dollars. A first-time offender convicted of second-degree theft usually would be required to post bail and then would be put on probation. However, because Brenda Vaughn tested positive for cocaine when she was arrested and because she was discovered to be seven months pregnant, the judge sentenced her to jail for the remainder of her pregnancy in order to protect her fetus. The judge "explicitly said that he was sentencing Vaughn to 'a long enough term in jail to be sure she would not be released

until her pregnancy was concluded.' There was no trial
or conviction on the allegations of illegal drug use."[26]

So far, we have seen law enforcement officials
working with doctors, social welfare workers, and judges
to effectively punish women for what they consider to
be inappropriate, and illegal, behavior for a pregnant
woman because it is harmful to her fetus. They have
depended upon the presence of controlled substances in
the blood and urine of newborns to prosecute women
for drug use.

Delivering Drugs through the Umbilical Cord

The methods discussed above are problematic
because, as evidenced by the explanation in Chapter 1,
the status of the fetus in the law is ambiguous. Is the
fetus a "minor" capable of having drugs delivered to it?
Is the fetus considered a person who can be the victim of
involuntary manslaughter or assault with a deadly
weapon? In an effort to avoid the complications
involved in trying to convict a woman of harming her
fetus by pre-natal drug use, prosecutors have developed
increasingly ingenious methods: because prosecutors do
not want to confront the fact that a fetus is not always
legally considered to be a person, they are claiming that
drugs are being delivered from mother to
fetus/newborn in the sixty to ninety seconds between
the time the that child is born and the time that the
umbilical cord is cut.

There are three cases that should be examined here.
Two of these were prosecuted by Tony Tague, the
District Attorney for Muskegon County, Michigan. The
first woman in Muskegon County to be arrested for
delivering drugs, in an amount of less than fifty grams,
to a minor through the umbilical cord was Kimberly

Ann Hardy, a twenty-three-year-old African-American woman on welfare. This is a felony in Michigan that carries a mandatory minimum jail term of one year, with the maximum sentence being twenty years. The other woman was Lynn Ellen Bremer who was thirty-six when she was arrested. Bremer is an attorney in Muskegon County; she is a white woman and a single mother. These two cases, when considered next to one another, support the assertion that drug use among pregnant women cuts across class lines and, while they highlight the similarities between these two women whose medical care was different, Hardy's and Bremer's cases demonstrate the impact of socio-economic conditions on drug use and pregnancy.

Kim Hardy told her doctor that she had used drugs during her pregnancy and her drug use was confirmed when toxicology tests were performed on her while she was in labor because she was considered to be a high risk pregnancy. (This means that she had received no pre-natal care and was delivering six to eight weeks early.)[7] Also, drug tests performed on her newborn revealed traces of *crack*. Bremer, on the other hand, had been receiving pre-natal care throughout her pregnancy; her obstetrician had known of her *cocaine* addiction for roughly five months and had not reported it. Bremer's obstetrician ordered the drug tests that were performed on her and her newborn baby. Neither woman had signed consent forms for the toxicology screenings yet, in both cases, the hospitals kept the newborns after the women were discharged; they performed drug tests and reported the findings to the Department of Social Services.

There is no law in Muskegon County that requires doctors to report positive drug tests to the social welfare organizations, but many do so out of a desire to see that both patients, woman and newborn, receive extra attention. Doctors report the findings to welfare workers in the hopes that a case worker will monitor a woman's drug use or her rehabilitation and will watch out for the welfare of the newborn.[28] This is often the way in which social service workers become involved in cases of pre-natal drug exposure.

Once the Department of Social Services became involved these women were served notices demanding their appearances at emergency hearings regarding the temporary removal of the newborns from maternal custody. (Again, the stated objective here was to protect the newborn infant from being placed in an abusive situation.) Both Hardy and Bremer lost custody of their newborn babies; Hardy's two other children, aged four years and eleven months were also removed from her custody despite the fact that neither appeared nor was proven to be neglected.

Both women entered thirty-day treatment programs while D.A. Tague filed suits against them. In neither case was the umbilical cord fluid tested for drugs despite the fact that the prosecution was relying on the delivery of drugs through this fluid from the mother to the newborn. Rather, the prosecution's cases rested solely on the results of the toxicology screens that were performed without consent; they claimed that drug testing was included in the general consent form that both Bremer and Hardy signed.[29]

Many people believe that the use of these tests as evidence in a criminal hearing violated the women's rights to privacy and against self-incrimination.[30] However, toxicology screenings do serve medical purposes; they are necessary in order for doctors to assess the condition of the newborn and to devise an effective treatment program.

The use of the drug test results as evidence in the criminal prosecution of women who use drugs during pregnancy is a complex issue: for the medical care of both the woman and the newborn toxicology information can be essential to physicians. It is also possible to see these tests as violations of privacy and as a segue to greater invasions into the lives of pregnant women. Alcohol, which is legal, can be detected as well; if drug tests are accepted as evidence in child abuse and neglect cases, the possibility of the criminalization of alcohol consumption during pregnancy is created. These are the kinds of invasions that civil libertarians and feminists fear because they threaten pregnant women's rights to autonomous behavior and subject them to societally defined standards of behavior.

These two Michigan examples raise another issue. Most of the women who have been prosecuted are like Kimberly Hardy; they are poor women of color who depend on public assistance. Lynn Bremer is the exception. She had adequate pre-natal care, she could have had access to drug treatment had she wanted it, but she didn't. So, poverty, or lack of access to care, is not the only problem underlying the use of drugs by pregnant women.

Lynn Bremer was addicted to cocaine and that was her most compelling concern; she was unwilling to give up her habit despite the fact that she was aware of the harmful effects of her drug use on her fetus. Despite the fact that Bremer's case may not inspire sympathy, she should not be criminally prosecuted for her addiction to cocaine. First of all, addiction is a disease, not a crime, and it has been recognized as such in both legal and medical forums. Criminalizing addiction will not encourage women, or men, to seek out treatment but rather force them to hide their addictions from health care providers, family members, and friends if admitting addiction carries the burden of possible prosecution.

Secondly, Bremer should not be held liable simply because she had the means to avoid exposing her fetus to drugs in utero. The prosecution of women like Lynn Bremer singles out pregnant addicts and treats them as criminals because their addiction has a direct, physiological impact on another individual. If women like Lynn Bremer are considered guilty simply because they have the options that women like Kim Hardy do not have then women of all ethnicities and socio-economic backgrounds are at risk of losing the freedom to treat themselves first and their fetuses second.

Both Hardy and Bremer have successfully completed drug treatment programs. Overcoming their addictions, was not enough, though, to cause Tague to drop the criminal charges against these women. However, on April 2, 1991, a Michigan appeals court ruled that Kimberly Hardy could not be forced to stand trial on charges of drug trafficking for delivering drugs to her fetus through the umbilical cord. (This decision overturned an earlier, lower court decision that Hardy could in fact be tried for violating the Michigan drug trafficking laws.) The decision explained that the legislators had never intended for the statute to be applied in this way when it was enacted.

When that decision was handed down, the state appeals court was the highest level court to rule on the question of the criminal prosecution of women who use drugs during pregnancy. According to Howard Simon, executive director of the Civil Liberties Union in Michigan, "[The] decision should effectively put an end to a vicious and counterproductive prosecutorial tactic," explaining that these prosecutions drive women away from treatment and pre-natal care.[31]

District Attorney Tague rallied by appealing the decision to the Michigan Supreme Court. For him, the debate over the validity of the criminality of drug use during pregnancy was not over; "This is a major health care crisis, and we must use whatever means we can to reach a solution. . . . When the war on drugs is making casualties out of newborn children, it requires action."[32] The Simon and Tague statements sum up the bottom line thinking of both advocates and opponents of criminalization. Finally, in June 1991 the Michigan Supreme Court upheld the appeals court decision, citing the same reason: The law that made drug trafficking to children a felony was not intended to criminalize the behavior of women during pregnancy.[33] The charges against Lynn Bremer were also dismissed: In February 1991, the Eaton County Circuit Court judge presiding over the case said that the suit violated Bremer's right to privacy "by intruding into her relationship with her fetus without a compelling reason to do so," and to due process because "she was not notified that the [drug trafficking] law could apply to her."[34] For now, no convictions have been obtained yet, but Tony Tague's efforts continue.

Florida is another state that has been testing the waters with regard to criminalization. The first woman to be convicted under a drug trafficking statute of delivering a controlled substance to a minor through her umbilical cord was Jennifer Johnson of Sanford, Florida. In the summer of 1989, Johnson, a twenty-three-year-old African-American woman, was sentenced to fourteen years of probation and one year of house arrest, to be served in a drug rehabilitation facility. The conditions of her probation were extremely specific: aside from being required to perform 200 hours of community service, Johnson is required to enter an intense pre-natal care program if she becomes pregnant again, she is forbidden to use drugs or alcohol, to go to bars, and to spend time with people who use drugs or alcohol. These aspects of her behavior are subject to observance by her probation officer for fifteen years of her life.[35] Jennifer Johnson had informed her doctors, during labor, that she had used drugs during pregnancy. This information was later used against her to obtain a conviction. Jennifer Johnson appealed her case.

On Thursday, April 18, 1991, the Fifth District Court of Appeals in Daytona Beach, Florida became the first state appeals court to uphold the conviction of a woman charged with delivering drugs to a newborn through the umbilical cord. Despite the fact that the Florida state legislature had specifically decided to treat addiction during pregnancy as a health, not a legal problem,[36] this court endorsed this prosecution method. The three judge panel that delivered the opinion was comprised of two men and one woman. The woman dissented calling the notion of applying this statute to this situation "absurd" and explaining that the only way for Johnson to have avoided passing drugs to her infant via her umbilical cord once she was in labor would be to cut the umbilical cord *before* the baby was born (so that the drug contaminated fluids could not be passed in the instants between the time the baby is born and the cord is cut) which probably would have killed *both* Johnson and her baby.[37]

Fourteen public health and public interest groups filed amicus briefs in on behalf of Jennifer Johnson. Groups like the Committee on Ethics of the American College of Obstetricians and Gynecologists objected in this case because of the questionable methods employed by the district attorneys. First of all, prosecutions such as these could lead to the criminalization of noncompliance with medical advice.[38] Also, the notion that drugs can be passed through the umbilical cord in these few instants is scientifically difficult to prove. Dr. Ira Chasnoff of NAPARE agrees with the female judge in Florida, "good ethics and good law have to be based on good science and we just don't have [the] kind of data [necessary to prove the transfer of drugs through the umbilical in those few moments.]"[39] It is these kinds of challenges to the methods of prosecuting, in fact to the notion of prosecuting, women for using controlled substances during pregnancy that keep advocates of this reproductive restriction constantly re-evaluating and re-working their techniques.

Child Abuse and Neglect

As the campaign to regulate women's behavior during pregnancy by introducing the threat of criminal prosecution rages on, criminal child abuse and neglect has become the new hope of district attorneys around the country. One prosecutor explained, "This is not a case of law enforcement reaching in ... obtain information on drug use by a pregnant women; it is protection of a child from physical abuse."[40] Prosecutors have had great difficulty in convincing judges that it constitutes drug trafficking (there has been only one success, yet many failures). It should not constitute criminal child abuse. Women who use drugs during pregnancy are being convicted of a "new and independent crime" according to Lynn Paltrow, an attorney at the American Civil Liberties Union Reproductive Rights Project, "becoming pregnant while addicted to drugs ... the biological event of becoming pregnant transforms the woman from a drug user to a drug trafficker or child abuser."[41]

It is important to remember that saying women should not be criminally prosecuted for child abuse or neglect as a result of their drug use during pregnancy does not mean that women who are addicts should not be brought into the social welfare system to have their competency with regard to raising children evaluated. The idea that a woman who uses drugs during pregnancy will be an unsatisfactory parent is not ludicrous. But, involving child protective services in a way that protects a newborn infant from its mother's addiction and encourages the mother to seek treatment will not have the same impact as incarcerating the mother. The latter will be more likely to discourage women from entering into any relationship with the social welfare system while the former recognizes the value of both women and children and acknowledges their individual rights to care.

The notion of the pregnant drug user as a criminal child abuser has been tested in several states. One advantage in charging these women with child abuse or neglect as opposed to drug trafficking is that "judges and probation officials [can] be harsher on pregnant women [because of their ability to] use discretionary powers that are difficult to challenge."[42] Basing cases on violation of state child abuse and neglect laws allows prosecutors to avoid conflict with the Supreme Court ruling in *Roe v Wade* which says that the fetus is not a "person" for purposes of protection by the law.

One woman, Diane Pfannensteil of Laramie, Wyoming, was arrested and charged with child abuse when she arrived at a hospital emergency room to be treated for injuries inflicted by her abusive husband. While in the emergency room, Pfannensteil was tested for alcohol; she was then arrested in the emergency room, placed in jail, and charged with criminal child abuse for endangering her fetus. The judge who heard her case dismissed it on the ground that alcohol consumption during pregnancy did not constitute the probable cause necessary to continue the case against Pfannensteil; the effects of the alcohol were indeterminable at the time of arrest and prosecution, and years could pass before the effects of her drinking could be determined. The charges against her were eventually dropped.

Pfannensteil abused alcohol during her pregnancy but the situation involving women who use controlled substances during pregnancy, a category that includes illegal drugs such as crack, cocaine, or marijuana, as well as prescription drugs, is different because their newborns often have symptoms of drug exposure and/or withdrawal at birth; also the use of these drugs is punishable by law. Child abuse statutes do address parental drug use and/or abuse as justifiable causes to remove children from the custody of their parents.

In Kentucky, a thirty-three-year-old white woman, Connie Welch O'Neal, was arrested for possession of drug paraphernalia and percadin (to which she had been addicted for over fifteen years) in November of 1989. When she gave birth in December to a boy who was suffering from "neonatal abstinence syndrome" the charges against her were expanded to include criminal child abuse. O'Neal's defense focused on the fact that addiction is recognized as a disease, not a crime that should be punished. The jury found her guilty of all charges and sentenced her to five years in jail. Since her sentencing, O'Neal has requested treatment for her percadin addiction and has filed an appeal.

There are many isolated incidents of women being charged with child abuse or neglect for using drugs during pregnancy. And while examining them one at a time would provide a broad base of evidence for the claim that criminal prosecution is not the way to solve the problems of drug use during pregnancy, a lack of pre-natal care, and the rising number of babies being born exposed to drugs, a careful look at the trend in one state, South Carolina, will provide a more useful study because it encompasses all these dilemmas. In South Carolina, since August of 1989, eighteen women have been charged with either criminal child neglect or the distribution of drugs to a minor. All but one of these women is an African-American. In addition, three other women have had their children taken away from them through proceedings in Family Court, even though they have not been subject to criminal proceedings.[43]

Greenville, South Carolina appears to serve as the hub of the efforts aimed at punishing drug-using pregnant women for child abuse. Three examples: one twenty-year-old woman was sentenced to three-and-a-half years in prison on criminal child neglect charges because she used cocaine during her pregnancy. Another woman was sentenced to ten years in jail when the prosecution seized on reports that she had failed to complete drug treatment more than once. A fifteen-year-old woman *and her parents* were all charged with criminal neglect when the young woman's newborn tested positive for drugs.[44]

These women, a drug user, a drug addict, and a teenage mother, should be concerned primarily with getting help for themselves like drug treatment and birth control education rather than attempting to protect themselves from the state's desire to prosecute them for their disadvantages. These should also be the state's concerns; the criminal prosecutions use up many resources that could be redirected to help women and their newborns survive poverty and recover from addiction. Most of the women prosecuted in South Carolina do not have the resources to get treatment and or care. According to Lynn Paltrow in an article published in *Criminal Justice Ethics* , all of the recent prosecutions for child abuse and neglect are against poor

women, more than half of whom are women of color.[45]
Poor women's options are already limited by their socio-
economic status in society; why must the state further
restrict their choices rather than providing them with
care, treatment and education?

Luckily, not all state efforts have been as successful as
the ones in South Carolina; prosecutors have met with
the same objections in child abuse cases as they did in
drug trafficking and manslaughter cases: judges are
often unwilling to find that the fetus is entitled to
protection under these laws. Therefore, understanding
the criminal child abuse and neglect statutes, (that is
what constitutes "abuse" and "neglect,") helps us to
understand why this has become the new focus of the
advocates of the prosecution of drug-using pregnant
women. These statutes vary from state to state, and are
presently in the process of undergoing serious changes
to accommodate these prosecutions.

The New York Family Court Act of 1979[46] defines
"abuse" as "physical injury by other than accidental
means which causes or creates a substantial risk of
death, or serious or protracted disfigurement or
protracted impairment of the function of any body
organ . . . " (§1012 (e)(i)). It defines a neglected child as
one "whose physical, mental or emotional condition
has been impaired or is in imminent danger as a result
of the failure of his[/her] parents . . . to exercise a
minimum degree of care. . . . " (§1012(f)(i). Neglect can
also occur, according to the Act in the case of parents
"misusing a drug or drugs; or misusing alcoholic
beverages" (§1012 (f)(i)(A). With these definitions,
prosecutors' decision to charge women with child abuse
and neglect in order to obtain a conviction for pre-natal
drug use seems logical. These statutes were designed to
protect children from harm inflicted by their parents;

also, states already have set up channels through which
to guide child abuse and neglect cases.

However, the same obstacle prosecutors could not
overcome in drug trafficking cases exists here; these
statutes were not originally intended to protect fetuses.
This does not mean that judges are unwilling to find
that pre-natal drug use constitutes neglect or abuse, but
rather that every case is a gamble. Each judge is entitled
to apply the statutes as she/he sees fit. Therefore the
results have been inconsistent.

In Broward County, Florida, Cassandra Gethers was
charged with using drugs during her pregnancy, which
the state then construed as child abuse. The judge in her
case ruled that the fetus was not a legal person for
purposes of the Florida child abuse statute.[47] In two
other cases, both in New York, women were convicted
of child abuse when their newborns were discovered to
have been exposed to drugs *in utero*. One judge, in *In Re
Vanessa F.*, stated, "a newborn baby having withdrawal
symptoms is prima facie a neglected baby."[48] Another
case, *In Re Male R.*, provides an interesting twist: here
the judge found that a baby born with mild withdrawal
symptoms, due to maternal use of alcohol, cocaine and
barbituates during pregnancy, was in danger of being
neglected were he to be placed with his mother. Still the
court would not find that the effect of pre-natal behavior
was enough to find neglect.[49] What this means is that
the judge removed the child from the custody of his
mother because he feared what could happen if he did
not. Yet, he was unwilling to find the mother guilty of
having criminally neglecting her child. Both of these
cases were decided in the late 1970s.

More recently, in Nassau County, New York, a
Family Court judge ruled that a pregnant woman's drug
use or lack of pre-natal care could constitute neglect. In
his decision, the judge recognized the woman's right to

have an abortion, but said that once she had decided to carry to term, or the time for an abortion had passed, a child *in utero* was equivalent to a child ex utero in the type of protection afforded it with regard to child neglect.[50]

Cases of child abuse and neglect involve not only legal and judicial arms of state power, but also government organizations like the Department of Social Services, which often instigate and oversee these prosecutions. These social service organizations have become active participants in this campaign. In Los Angeles County, a positive urine test on a newborn infant is considered to be evidence of possible child abuse and requires that the infant be taken from its mother immediately.[51] The Nassau County Department of Social Services investigates any case in which a newborn tests positive for drugs, indicating that the mother has used drugs within the last seventy-two hours; these mothers are then charged with neglect, and can lose custody of their children immediately.[52]

LEGISLATORS: MAKING IT EASIER FOR THE DISTRICT ATTORNEYS AND THE JUDGES

These cases help to set the stage for the legislative overhaul that has taken place over the past two to three years in the area of child abuse and neglect. Many states have amended their codes to explicitly include the fetus as entitled to protection by the statutes. At least eleven states have enacted legislation designed to protect fetuses from abuse while they are *in utero*: Florida, California, Massachusetts, New Jersey, Illinois, Indiana, Oklahoma, New York, Nevada, Rhode Island, Minnesota, and Utah.

This legislation intends to criminalize the use of drugs and alcohol by pregnant women. Illinois, for example, amended its Juvenile Court Act to include infants born with controlled substances in their systems in the definition of a neglected minor. Other states have made similar changes in their definitions of children in need of services, or children who are being deprived. Other states, like New Jersey, have amended statutes so that they may be applied "on behalf of an unborn child . . . "[53] This section (§ 30:4c-11) of the New Jersey code can be applied so that the state can take custody of a child *in utero* if it feels that the woman's actions are endangering the fetus.[54] These changes in the law facilitate the process of obtaining a conviction for child abuse and neglect in these states, and enable states to take custody of newborns when they are born effected by controlled substances.

There are two possible courses of action that can be taken as a result of these legislative overhauls: First of all, the state can move in after a child is born to criminally prosecute the woman and remove the child from the custody of its mother. Secondly, some states can now access a fetus *in utero*, that is take custody of it before it is born, which effectively amounts to sentencing a woman to jail for the duration of her pregnancy to prevent her from abusing her fetus. The second option, which can now be applied in New Jersey, has the greatest potential to threaten women's freedom and autonomy. Because of statutes like this one, opponents of criminalization fear child abuse and neglect convictions; women can be put in jail because a state can take custody of an entity (that is traditionally not protected by law) which is growing inside of her. The notion that a fetus can be in the custody of a state while it is *in utero* is terrifying; a woman's life can be interrupted because the protection of her fetus takes priority over her freedom and her rights.

Other states, like Minnesota, have passed laws that make the flow of information between medical professionals and welfare agencies legal, and even mandatory in some cases. The Minnesota law requires that hospital officials report women who have, or are believed to have, used a controlled substance during pregnancy to a local welfare agency.[55]

In even bolder moves, state legislatures in Arizona, New Mexico, Rhode Island, Utah, and Michigan attempted, in 1983, to pass legislation equating the "criminally caused death of a fetus with manslaughter or homicide." Arkansas proposed a state constitutional amendment that would have made the state responsible for protecting "every unborn child from conception to birth."[56] These earlier attempts were apparently too bold, for most of them were blocked, and the efforts aimed at restructuring child abuse laws have been more successful both because they are not as extreme as these immature efforts, but also because the climate surrounding the issue of pre-natal drug exposure had warmed up. So far, nineteen states have passed laws that allow child abuse charges to be brought against a woman who gives birth to a child with illegal drugs in her/his bloodstream.[57]

Even national legislatures have become involved. Two bills were introduced in the 101st Congress. Senator Pete Wilson of California introduced the Child Abuse During Pregnancy Prevention Act of 1989 which called for the criminalization of such behavior. Compulsory treatment is also part of his program. The stated purpose of Senator Wilson's bill, which would amend the Public Health Service Act, is "to establish model projects concerning the effect of substance abuse on pregnant females, postpartum females and infants, and for other purposes." ... The other purposes appear to be to establish that "substance abuse by a pregnant woman is a form of child abuse ... " because "a woman who chooses to carry a pregnancy to term has a responsibility for the health and welfare of her child which *requires* that she refrain from substance abuse during her pregnancy" (emphasis added). This legislation also "finds" that drug testing of newborn infants is necessary to ensure that maternal substance abuse is "brought to the attention of the proper authorities."

Like Senator Bradley's bill discussed below, this bill allocates funds ($50,000,000 for fiscal year 1990) to be granted, at the discretion of the Director of the Office of Substance Abuse, to states which can meet the requirements set forth in the legislation. Eligibility for a grant is contingent upon devising a comprehensive plan to prevent maternal substance abuse during pregnancy; the plan must include preventive outreach and education, provision for penalizing women who give birth to substance addicted infants, and treatment for both mother and child. Any state applying for federal grants under this program must be willing to agree to a plan that authorizes health care providers to report substance abusing mothers to the "authorities," to agree that giving birth to an infant exposed to controlled substances in the womb constitutes child abuse, and to agree that it is a crime punishable by "three years of mandatory rehabilitation in a custodial setting" in addition to probation. This legislation, on the surface appears to be aimed at providing care for women and children, but in fact makes prosecution and punishment a priority.

The other bill introduced was S.708 which Bill Bradley of New Jersey presented to the Senate in April 1989. This bill, the Healthy Birth Act of 1989 was designed "[t]o amend title V of the Social Security Act to promote the integration and coordination of services for pregnant women and infants to prevent and reduce infant mortality and morbidity." This legislation would allocate $661,000,000 for fiscal year 1990 to establish programs that would enable pregnant women to obtain better pre-natal care. The bill also sets up a system of requirements that must be met in order to receive federal funds under this program; these include increased access to information about pregnancy and to pre-natal care facilities. The programs would be developed and monitored by the National Commission to Prevent Infant Mortality. Both medicaid and the special supplemental food program for women, infants and children (WIC) would be involved in determining the eligibility of state proposed programs. The exact terms of this legislation will be discussed in Chapter 3 as part of a discussion on advocacy. Senator Bradley's bill, unlike Senator Wilson's, does not endorse the criminal prosecution of women who use drugs during pregnancy; rather it wisely focuses on identifying and solving the underlying causes. But, this is only one effort.

Advancements in the late 1970s and early 1980s in the fields of neonatology and perinatology coupled with an explosion of anti-abortion (pro-life) sentiment, caused a campaign for fetal rights to emerge into the mainstream. The early results were forced obstetrical interventions. As the interest in the fetus intensified and infant mortality increased, greater efforts were made to protect fetuses and ensure that they were born healthy. The criminal prosecution of women who use drugs during pregnancy was the result of these societal forces.

The examples discussed in this chapter illustrate that there are many causes of the crisis of pre-natal drug exposure that are more deeply embedded in society than drug use among pregnant women. These are poverty, addiction, inadequate pre-natal care, and insufficient drug treatment opportunities. Chapter 3 will examine these causes and explain why it is essential that fetal rights not become the sole focus of any effort to reduce the number of babies exposed prenatally to drugs. Women, their care, treatment, and rights, need to be taken into account for a complete solution to be devised.

NOTES

[1] This theory was confirmed in a telephone interview with Dr. Isabelle Wilkins, Assistant Professor of Obstetrics and Gynecology at the University of Texas in Houston.

[2] V.Kolder at al, 1202-1206.

[3] Gallagher, 62.

[4] Ibid, 64.

[5] For the same reason, The Supreme Court in 1973 agreed to hear *Roe v Wade* despite the fact that Jane Roe was no longer pregnant. Pregnancies last only nine months which, given the overburdened judicial system in this country, is not always enough time to reach the proper judicial channels.

[6] Susan Edmiston, "Here Come the Pregnancy Police," *Glamour*, August 1990, 204.

[7] Jefferson v Griffin Spalding County Hospital Authority, 274 S.E. 2d 451 (Ga. 1981).

[8] Gallagher, 66.

[9] Amana, 25-6.

[10] Robertson, "Procreative Liberty and the Control of Conception, Pregnancy, and Childbirth," *Virginia Law Review* 69 (1983) 405, 437-438.

[11] Lynn Paltrow, "When Becoming Pregnant Is a Crime," *Criminal Justice Ethics*, Winter/Spring 1990, 41-47.

[12] *New York Times* 9 January 1989, I, 1: 1.

[13] Angela Bonavoglia, "The Ordeal of Pamela Rae Stewart," *Ms.* ,July/Aug. 1987, 93.

[14] Ibid, 92.

[15] Paltrow, 42.

[16] Edmiston, 204.

[17] Jan Hoffman, "Pregnant, Addicted and Guilty," *New York Times Magazine*, 19 August 1990, 35.

[18] Dorothy E. Roberts, "The Future of Reproductive Choice for Poor Women and Women of Color," *Women's Rights Law Reporter*, 12 No. 2 (1990): 66.

[19] Dorothy E. Roberts, "Mother as Martyr," *Essence* , May 1991, 140.

[20] Both the ACLU and I would like to point out that this figure is almost identical to the figure regarding court-ordered obstetrical interventions performed on women of color.

[21] Roberts, "Mother as Martyr," 140.

[22] Susan LaCroix, "Jailing Mothers for Drug Abuse," *The Nation*, 1 May 1989, 585.

[23] Andrea Sachs, "Here Come the Pregnancy Police," *Time*, 22 May 1989, 104.

[24] Gallagher, 67.

[25] Sharon Begley, "The Troubling Question of Fetal Rights," *Newsweek*, 8 December 1986, 87.

26 American Civil Liberties Union memorandum, "State by State Case Summary of Criminal Prosecutions Against Pregnant Women" 29 October 1990, 3.

27 Hoffman, p. 35.

28 In an April 15, 1990 telephone interview with Dr. Isabelle Wilkins, an Assistant Professor of Obstetrics and Gynecology at the University of Texas who specializes in neonatology, I learned that many doctors who deal with public assistance patients or patients without insurance report positive toxicology tests to welfare workers, but not to law enforcement officials.

29 Hoffman, 34.

30 Ibid. See my discussion of the Supreme Court's unwillingness to force a criminal suspect to subject her/himself to medical tests to provide evidence that could be used against her/him in Chapter 1.

31 Isabel Wilkerson, "Woman Cleared After Drug Use in Pregnancy," *New York Times*, 3 April 1991, A,15.

32 Ibid.

33 "Michigan Court Backs Mother in Drug Case," *New York Times*, June 18, 1991, B,7: 2.

34 "Judge Drops Charges of Delivering Drugs to an Unborn Baby," *New York Times*, February 5, 1991, B;6: 4.

35 American Civil Liberties Union, "State by State Case Summary of Criminal Prosecutions Against Pregnant Women," 29 October 1990, p. 6.

36 Tamar Lewin, "Court in Florida Upholds Conviction for Drug Delivery by Umbilical Cord," *New York Times*, 20 April 1991, I, 6: 4.

37 Ibid.

38 Paltrow, 45.

39 Hoffman, 36.

40 "Punishing Pregnant Addicts: Debate, Dismay, No Solution," *New York Times* 10 September 1989, IV, 5: 1.

41 Paltrow, 42.

42 Ted Gest, "The Pregnancy Police on Patrol," *U.S. News and World Report*, 6 February 1989, 50.

43 American Civil Liberties Union memorandum, "State by State Case Summary of Criminal Prosecutions Against Pregnant Women." October 29, 1990: 12.

44 Ibid.

45 Paltrow, 42.

46 I chose New York State as an example because I am writing and living in New York, also many of the child abuse cases I discovered in my research took place in New York State. Many of the treatment programs I will examine in Chapter 3 are also in New York. Most child abuse statutes are derived in some form from the Children's Bureau Model Act which defines abuse as "serious physical injury or injuries inflict by other than accidental means."

47 American Civil Liberties Union memorandum, "State by State Case Summary of Criminal Prosecutions Against Pregnant Women." October 29, 1990: 5.

48 351 N. Y. S. 2d 337, 340.

49 Amana, 7..See also 422 N. Y. S. 2d 819, 822.

[50] Tamar Lewin, "When Courts Take Charge of the Unborn," *New York Times,* 9 January 1989, A, 1: 1.

[51] Ibid.

[52] Ibid.

[53] Amana, 13.

[54] Johnson, 604.

[55] Paltrow, 45

[56] Begley, 88.

[57] James Willwerth, "Should We Take Away Their Kids?" *Time* 13 May 1991, 62-63

III

Causes and Effects

Very little is being done to combat the underlying problems which have sparked this campaign against pregnant women who use drugs. Health care providers, law enforcement officials, welfare workers, and legislators are legitimately concerned with the rising rate of babies born disadvantaged by pre-natal exposure to controlled substances. Yet, so far all efforts have been aimed at the surface level; the least expensive, least disruptive method is for the criminal justice system to point its finger at the mothers.

But, many factors (drug use among pregnant women is not the seminal problem) have combined to produce this crisis; and society's commitment to solving these riddles is uneven. The use of drugs in this society is being addressed: The War on Drugs is being waged on all levels of government. Millions of dollars every year are allocated to stamping out illegal drug use. But, resources also need to be directed at the other causes of this crisis like the lack of adequate pre-natal care for women (especially those dependent on public assistance) and the lack of drug treatment facilities for pregnant drug users and addicts. Rather than ostracizing and blaming pregnant women for circumstances often beyond their control, and rather than sending them to jail because they are victims of diseases which have

ravaged all sectors of society (poverty and addiction),
federal, state, and local governments should be focusing
their efforts on providing care for women and children.
The criminal prosecution of women who use drugs
during pregnancy can only burden two already
inadequate systems—the criminal justice system and the
foster care system—while failing to attack the roots of
the problem, namely poverty, drug dependency, and
inadequate health care.

It is necessary to have some sense of the
overwhelming impact of drugs and insufficient pre-
natal care and drug treatment programs to understand
why the struggle has been reduced to creating a
competition for protection and resources between
mothers and children. Hundreds of thousands of babies
are born each year addicted to controlled substances. The
majority of women in this country receive inadequate
pre-natal care, regardless of their relationship with
drugs.

There are risks involved in driving a wedge between
mothers and newborns, especially for women. All
women who are capable of bearing children are in
jeopardy because any program that criminalizes the
behavior of pregnant women because they are pregnant
women can only lead to an infringement on the rights
of women as a group. All women can be seen as
potential mothers and therefore subject to societal
restrictions on behavior that would not be tolerated by
other groups. The threat of a "slippery slope" on which
women will slide to the bottom of society's list of
priorities is real. Only a program designed to
acknowledge and respond to the breadth of causes that
exist here can have the desired effect: healthier babies
and healthier, drug free moms.

The agenda that is being advanced today which
places fetuses above women and children is seen by

some[1] as "a cheap flashy way to look like you're doing something about a difficult problem when in fact you're not . . . [because] the criminal justice system can't pass a law to make poverty go away." George J. Annas, a professor of Health Law at the Boston University School of Medicine, is not the only one who sees the campaign for fetal rights as being an insufficient response to a national health crisis. Ira Chasnoff of NAPARE calls it a " . . . short-term, knee-jerk reaction . . . caused by [so much] frustration that people are beginning to lash out at the group with the least defenses—women, especially the minority poor."[2]

The women who are most affected by the lack of pre-natal care and drug treatment are women who are dependent on Medicaid for health care. They are also the women most ravaged by the effects of crack cocaine. They are the women who give birth in public hospitals. Poor women are the women least likely to have choices; for example, is abortion really an option for a drug addicted pregnant woman whose only source of health insurance is Medicaid, which does not cover abortion?

A solution to this problem is not one dimensional. This crisis can not be abated simply by throwing women in jail where they are deprived of the freedoms that can harm or help their fetuses. The causes are numerous; the mere fact that some believe that by punishing women, babies will be born healthier indicates that the roots of the problem lie in the *moral*, as well as the legal, social, and medical realms of our society. Women can not be held responsible for the welfare of the next generation (which is what the advocates of criminal prosecution are pushing for) if they do not have the support systems necessary to safeguard the health of their fetuses. Putting women behind bars will not solve the problem. Consider the root causes.

THE CAUSES

The government has decided to address the issue of an estimated 375,000 newborns born in one year exposed to illegal drugs.[3] There are three basic underlying problems that the current agenda of criminal prosecution does not address: drug use among pregnant women, inadequate pre-natal care, and a lack of drug treatment facilities for pregnant women and poor women. Because the government has chosen to address only the end result of a huge, multi-faceted crisis that touches all sectors of society, a solution does not seem to be forthcoming. Their punitive methods risk three possible effects: the criminalization of addiction, the exclusion of women from a successful solution as a result of the focus on the fetus, and the detrimental effect that the criminalization of drug use during pregnancy could have on the rights of women as members of society.

Drug Use Among Pregnant Women

In 1988, NAPARE conducted a survey of thirty-six hospitals across the United States. The survey covered 154,856 births; it was discovered that eleven percent of the mothers had used illegal drugs (including marijuana, cocaine, PCP, heroin and amphetamines) during their pregnancies.[4]

The House Select Committee on Children, Youth, and Families held several hearings in 1990 to address the crisis of "Women, Infants and Perinatal Substance Abuse." The committee reported several other studies that had been performed around the country, illustrating how widespread perinatal drug use is.

Individual localities have also conducted surveys of mothers and newborns; Pinellas County, Florida surveyed 715 pre-natal or postpartum women, and fifteen percent of them tested positive for substance abuse. The Pinellas County sampling showed no socio-economic differences among the women.[5]

In 1989 a survey of eight cities discovered that an estimated 9,000 babies were born exposed to illicit drugs. These 9,000 babies and the complications they will suffer because of their perinatal drug exposure will cost an estimated $500,000,000 between the time they are born and their fifth birthdays.[6]

The House Subcommittee hearings also provided a number of profiles of substance abusing women. A 1989 hospital survey performed in Rhode Island discovered that 7.5 % of the women involved in the study tested positive for at least one drug. In Rhode Island, women on public aid were four times as likely to test positive for drugs; cocaine use was more common among women of color, used public insurance, were living in "poverty," and/or delivered at a regional perinatal center.

Other characteristics of mothers who give birth to babies who test positive for controlled substances are malnutrition, unplanned pregnancies, sexually transmitted diseases (STDs), and little to no pre-natal care.[7]

Infant mortality has been on the rise in the past few years and most sources agree that drug use by pregnant women has contributed largely to the declining condition of newborn babies. But experts who push the question one step further have discovered that inadequate nutrition, poor education, teenage pregnancy, and smoking, drinking and drug use during pregnancy have all been significant factors; these causes however *are* *not* the root of the problem. The prosecution of women for drug use during pregnancy is not going to solve the problems of inadequate pre-natal care and drug treatment programs for pregnant women in this country. The number of babies born exposed to drugs every year should be sparking a debate, but not a debate about how to punish women for their role; rather it should be a debate about how to help women help themselves and their infants.

Lack of Pre-Natal Care

An estimated 74,000 women a year receive no pre-natal care at all; 154,00 women a year get care only late in third trimester of pregnancy. Twenty-five percent of all women aged eighteen to twenty-four have no medical coverage for pre-natal care or delivery.[8] One article stated that more than one quarter of "women of reproductive age" have no insurance to cover maternity care and two-thirds of these have no health insurance at all.[9] Twelve Counties in California have no facilities willing to treat pregnant women on Medi-Cal (the state health-care program for the poor).[10] At Boston City Hospital, eighty percent of mothers surveyed who used cocaine or crack during their pregnancy received no pre-natal care at all. In New York City, women who use cocaine are seven times less likely than women who did not to have received no pre-natal care. These statistics are staggering; how are women who do not receive pre-natal care supposed to be able to care for themselves and their fetuses? How are they supposed to know of the damage that drugs and alcohol cause to their fetuses? And even if they did know, how are they supposed to treat themselves? These women have no access to medical care during pregnancy.

The reason that a lack of pre-natal care can be seen as an underlying cause of this crisis is that without pre-natal care women who are pregnant and addicted have no interaction with the health care system at all. If the government were really concerned with improving the health of women during pregnancy, they should target their energies at deconstructing the barriers to care. Providing obstetric care yields an opportunity to treat women and refer them to treatment programs. If women were to receive adequate pre-natal care, that included regular visits to an obstetrician, their progress could be monitored; someone would be following up on the development of the drug addiction as it impacted the fetus as well as the mother. In her statement before the House Select Committee mentioned above, Sheila Blume, the Medical Director at South Oaks Hospital in Amityville, New York, explained, "Pregnancy is the best time to treat . . . a chemically dependant woman. The incentive to have the best healthiest possible infant is a tremendous motivator for treatment. Throwing such a woman in jail where she will get no incentive . . . is the opposite of what should be happening."[11]

Federal maternal and child-health block grants dropped from $478 million in 1983 to $399 million in 1984 alone.[12] A single woman living alone must have an income below the federal poverty level to qualify for medicaid in most states; in 1986, the cut off income was eighty-eight dollars a month. In twenty states a pregnant woman living in a two-salary household cannot receive Medicaid coverage for pre-natal care regardless of how much income is generated by those two salaries.[13]

The Committee on Alcohol and Drug Dependent Women and Their Children's (CADDWC) statement on access to health care services claims that $5,000.00 is the average annual income eligibility ceiling for Medicaid. The report goes on to point out that 44% of obstetrical and gynecological care providers do not accept Medicaid patients because reimbursement systems are ineffective. The CADDWC report also listed lack of day-care facilities, geographic inaccessibility, and poor communication between doctors and patients due to language and socio-economic differences as barriers to care for poor pregnant women.[14]

Recently (March 1991) three publicly funded clinics closed in New York. These clinics, which served about 10,000 women were shut down as a result of federal budget cuts. These clinics provided women in Manhattan, Brooklyn, and Queens with routine examinations, counseling, birth control prescriptions, diaphragms, Pap smears and obstetrical referrals. The women who used these clinics are now without gynecological care. In addition, in the same month, Planned Parenthood of New York City discontinued these services at their Manhattan office due to financial difficulties. An article in the *New York Times* called "Close of Clinics Rocks Poor Women," explained that the federal budget for family planning was $162 million in 1980; by 1990 it was down to $144 million.[15]

The government's commitment to stamping out infant mortality does not extend to providing women with the attention necessary to have healthy children. Consider President Bush's campaign to reduce infant mortality by diverting funds from the already scarce health programs that serve pregnant women and poor children; he proposed taking $33.7 million from the Maternal and Child Health Block Grant to wage a campaign against infant mortality in 10 localities. The Secretary of Health and Human Services, Dr. Louis W. Sullivan justified the proposal by saying, "that it would be much more effective when concentrated in 10 target areas than when spread around the country, as it is in the Maternal and Child Health Block Grant. . . . "[16]

Luckily, Congress rejected the Bush proposal and instead allocated $25 million "new" dollars to combat infant mortality rather than take it from the already inadequate Block Grants. However, even though Congress was unable to say where the money would come from; at least they are recognizing the need to address the concerns of both women and fetuses/newborns. Still, if there is no way for these women to get pre-natal care, how can they be held responsible for the effects of their behavior?

Lack of Drug Treatment

Pregnant women who use drugs are in even worse shape. Drug treatment programs are not geared towards the treatment of women and they are not equipped to handle pregnant addicts. Most do not even accept pregnant women into their programs because of the liability associated with high-risk pregnancies. There appears to be a consensus among the majority of politicians, welfare workers, medical professionals, and law enforcement officials that criminal prosecution of women who use drugs during pregnancy is a wrong-headed approach to the problem; existing drug treatment facilities are simply not sufficient enough to satisfy the demand. Anne O'Reilly, the Director of Family and Children's Services for the San Francisco Department of Social Services testified before the House Select Committee, "If these mothers were walking away from treatment, I might feel differently. But they're not walking away from treatment—they're walking away from waiting lists."[17] Janet Gallagher is quoted as saying that laws that attempt to force addicted women to get treatment are "ludicrous" because so few treatment programs exist.[18]

Most people would agree that getting women into treatment programs is at least a step in the right direction; even attempts to force pregnant addicts into treatment can be rationalized by explaining that it helps both the woman and the fetus. However, requiring pregnant drug users to get treatment or be prosecuted without providing adequate facilities puts women in an impossible position.

A survey of hospitals in large metropolitan areas conducted in 1989 found that two-thirds had no place to refer substance abusing pregnant women. Dr. Wendy Chavkin at the Columbia University School of Public Health performed a study of drug treatment programs in New York City. She found that fifty-four percent of the programs refused to admit pregnant women; sixty-seven percent denied access to pregnant women on Medicaid; and eighty-seven percent turned away women who were pregnant, on Medicaid, and addicted to crack. Less than half of these programs arranged pre-natal care when they did accept pregnant women; only two arranged child care. These programs do not provide child care despite the fact that the National Institute for Drug Abuse (NIDA) research shows that this lack "effectively precludes" women from getting drug addiction treatment.[19]

In California, there are only five full time drug treatment programs that accept women; each of them has waiting lists up to six months long.[20] Atlanta has only two programs that offer specialized programs for women. In Butte County, California, the District Attorney, Michael Ramsey, announced in 1988 that county hospitals would begin testing all newborns suspected of being exposed to drugs while *in utero*, and that the results would be used to prosecute the mother. Ramsey said that the women would have a choice between drug treatment and ninety days in jail. But the facts are that Butte County's drug treatment facilities cannot accommodate these women; waiting lists are up to six months long and the facilities are inaccessible by public transportation.[21]

Butte County provides an example of the impracticality of giving women a "choice" between treatment and incarceration; that choice just does not exist. Ramsey's proposal seems to suggest that women who want treatment will be able to get it, but he ignores the fact that the resources cannot accommodate his plan. Lynn Paltrow of the ACLU points out that according to the American Bar Association Standards for Criminal Justice, "prosecutors should be familiar with the resources of social agencies. . . . " in applying criminal statutes and trying criminal cases.[22] The inadequacy of the drug treatment facilities around this country is no secret, especially to prosecutors who are aware of the prevalence of drug use among pregnant women. If Ramsey and other law enforcement officials want to give pregnant addicts a chance to help themselves and save their fetuses then they should work to ensure the expansion of drug treatment facilities that will meet with the demands of the crisis. Otherwise, they really are condemning these women to jail without giving them any other option except to remain outside the systems that otherwise could help them.

The shortage of drug treatment facilities for pregnant addicts is bad enough for women who can afford to pay for private care, but for women dependent upon public assistance the situation is even worse. Medicaid only covers seventeen days of the standard twenty-eight day treatment program. Medicaid is also selective in the kinds of drug treatment it will cover; heroin addicts can get what little coverage there is, but Medicaid will not provide subsidies for crack addiction treatment.

Pregnant drug-using women need to be encouraged to get help for themselves if society is intent on making women solely responsible for the care of children. Treatment programs are not designed to accommodate the special needs of women. As Dr. Chavkin's survey points out, pre-natal care and child care are not generally available to women addicts despite the fact that the provision of these services would make drug treatment a much more realistic possibility for pregnant addicts.

Drug treatment facilities discriminate against pregnant women. While it is true that many of them lack pre-natal or obstetric services, they are still in violation of federal laws which prohibit discrimination on the basis of sex *and* pregnancy.[23] These facilities cite a concern for the health of the fetus when they deny access to pregnant women, (and a fear of legal liability for any damage suffered by a patient's fetus) but this reasoning is faulty: First, it is possible for a woman to detox without harming her fetus if she is monitored properly. Second, the doctrine of informed consent should protect the facility if they advise the women of the risks involved before treatment begins. And last, the ravages of drugs on fetal health are widely known, given this, any "concern for the fetus" that keeps women out of drug treatment facilities *because* they are pregnant is questionable.[24] A woman's drug use *will* harm her fetus, while her drug rehabilitation, which will improve the health of the woman, could also save her fetus.

In California, there are 366 publicly-funded drug treatment programs; sixty-seven of them treat women, and of those only sixteen can accommodate a woman and her dependent children. Ohio has sixteen women's recovery centers; only two of them provide care for the patients' children.[25] New York City has only one treatment facility where mothers and their small

children can live together. This program, called Mothers
and Babies Off Narcotics (MABON) also provides pre-
natal care for pregnant women. New Haven,
Connecticut also has one such program: Crossroads.
Officials at this facility estimate that 750 women in New
Haven used illicit drugs during pregnancy in one year.
They also point out that there are only two publicly
funded treatment programs in Connecticut that accept
pregnant women; they can accommodate only twenty-
five women at a time and they each have a two month
waiting list.

In 1990, Congress mandated that states spend at least
10% of the federal Alcohol, Drug Abuse and Mental
Health Services block grant on the development of
prevention and treatment programs for alcohol and
drug dependent women, especially pregnant women.
Most states have not complied.[26] How are pregnant
addicts supposed to avoid prosecution if they have no
opportunity for treatment?

Reed Tuckson, M.D., Senior Vice President for
Programs at the March of Dimes Foundation,stated at
the congressional hearing, "Beyond the Stereotypes",

> When we look at our responses to this
> problem [of perinatal substance abuse], it is
> clear that we do not have enough pre-
> natal care, period. . . . We do not have
> enough drug treatment programs by
> several orders of magnitude.
>
> What is even more frustrating is that
> there is no relationship between the drug
> programs and the pre-natal care programs.
>
> I don't understand how we ever get into
> discussions about separating the baby out
> from the mother. It's all connected, the

> mother's pre-natal care is connected to the
> drug abuse care, the child is connected *in
> utero* to the mother. Its all one thing that
> needs to be coordinated and unified.[27]

THE EFFECTS

In addition to the fact that the criminal prosecution
of women who use drugs during pregnancy as a
solution to the growing crisis of drug use among
pregnant women does not respond adequately and fairly
to the pre-existing conditions (inadequate pre-natal care
and drug treatment), it also ignores the possible effects
that it could have upon women and children. It would
effectively lead to the criminalization of addiction, to a
focus on the fetus as the sole entity worth saving from
the ravages of drug addiction in pregnant women, and
to a potentially devastating infringement on the rights
of women.

The Criminalization of Addiction

There is a marked lack of treatment for drug
addiction for all addicts, male and female; however,
women addicts face additional gender-based obstacles in
receiving treatment. If prosecutors continue to treat
women as criminals for their drug use during
pregnancy, and if they become increasingly successful as
time passes, then pregnant drug addicts will have to
confront yet another obstacle: the criminalization of
their addiction by society.

While it is true that drug use in pregnant women
cuts across class lines, low-income women and minority

women are comprising more and more of the population ravaged by substance abuse. Studies have shown that seventy percent of drug addicted women have been victims of violence by their partners or spouses. Fifteen percent of the women surveyed had been raped as children and twenty-one percent had been raped as adults.[28]

A second obstacle that makes it more difficult for women than men to receive drug treatment is that women, as the primary care takers in this society, often have children to care for. Drug treatment centers do not provide women with child care and this, as pointed out above, creates a barrier between women and treatment. In his testimony before the House Select Committee, Dr. Alan I. Trachtenberg, Medical Director at Bay Area Addiction, Research and Treatment and the Family Addiction Center for Education and Treatment, points out that, "addiction, along with many other diseases, is a public health consequence of oppression and poverty. He goes on to say that, "[m]ost influential people in our society seem to have little interest in an addicted woman until she becomes pregnant. . . . After delivery, society again loses interest in the woman, except in her role as a potentially unfit mother."[29]

The ways in which drug treatment programs are structured and implemented does not take into consideration the special needs of women. "Most drug and alcoholism treatment models are based on premises about drug use and societal roles that are predominantly male-oriented."[30] It is also true that women are less encouraged by society, friends, and family to participate in treatment because of their role as care-taker to men and children in our society. Given these already daunting obstacles, women dependant on drugs certainly do not need the additional burden of the criminalization of their addiction. Why should women addicts be punished by the law while men addicts are simply encouraged to get treatment? Women certainly will not be able to overcome their addictions from inside an already over-crowded jail, most of which do not provide drug treatment anyway.[31] The criminalization of addiction for pregnant women (and all women with childbearing capabilities) will push women further away from the drug treatment system rather than frighten them in to getting treatment. To wit, Kim Hardy, who was accused of delivering drugs to her fetus through her umbilical cord, said that she would not have told her doctor about her drug use if she had known what would happen to her.[32] As so many experts have said, women will not get treatment at the cost of their freedom.[33] Who would?

Focus on the Fetus

Society's interest in women addicts intensifies when they become pregnant; this belies an interest in women's care that is dependent on their role as childbearer. This focus on the fetus marginalizes women. Lynn Paltrow explains that, "historically women have been held to a higher moral standard and forced to sacrifice their civil rights and civil liberties because of their childbearing capacity."[34]

The fetal rights campaign which has recently focused on drug and alcohol use among pregnant women is seen by many as being "inconsistent and fitful"; it has changed its focus from forced obstetrical interventions discussed in Chapter 2 to the prosecution of drug-using pregnant women.[35] The campaign for fetal rights, which is part of the motivation behind the criminal prosecution of women who use drugs during pregnancy, enables the fetus to enjoy a privileged status in society, above that of both women and children. Many of the consequences of the focus on the fetus already can be seen in society: the Webster decision which created the potential for restrictions on a woman's right to procure an abortion, forced obstetrical interventions, and the criminal prosecution pregnant addicts. Feminists and civil libertarians fear even greater infringements on the rights of women in this society if the campaign for fetal rights is allowed to continue to keep society focused on the unborn.

Foster Care

In devoting so many resources to the protection of the fetus, fetal rights activists are overburdening already inadequate foster care systems that were designed to protect children. In the cases examined in Chapter 2 , the women who were prosecuted lost custody of their newborns on the basis of positive drug tests. A positive toxicology screen should not always lead to the separation of a woman from her child because it is not adequate to distinguish between a one time user and an addict; and it is contrary to laws that require "preventive services" be provided before removal in an effort to keep families together.[36]

There is an acute shortage of foster care in this country, especially in urban areas ravaged by poverty and drug use. Tim Willwerth's article in *Time* entitled, "Should We Take Away Their Kids?," argues that removing children from their mothers can be more detrimental than attempting to keep the family intact. Newborns often become wards of the state living in hospitals for months. This institutional care can lead to a "failure to thrive," a medical term for babies who do not gain enough weight to survive and who fail to develop.[37]

Both New York and Los Angeles, two cities hit hardest by the crack epidemic, have backed away form the "seize the kid" approach because their systems are completely overloaded. Policies that mandate the removal of newborns because of a positive toxicology screen "put the state in the position of destroying families as the quick and easy answer to the drug epidemic," said Susan Demers of the New York State Department of Social Services.[38] When you consider the effect that prosecuting women for using drugs can have on the newborn it becomes clear why a sound solution to this crisis must try to preserve the dignity of both the mother and the child by addressing the underlying causes.

The Slippery Slope

The obstetrical interventions and prosecutions discussed in Chapter 2 may only be the beginning of the fetal rights campaign; women's rights to care and to autonomy are currently being challenged, but what if they are eliminated? When resources such as money and time, are channeled away from women toward fetuses, fetuses gain at the expense of women. If this divergence continues, the consequences for women could be irreparable.

Fetal rights has already led to forced medical procedure, and criminal prosecution of pregnant women. Society's desire to protect the unborn, or rather to guarantee healthy newborns has also spilled over into the work place; women have been deprived of jobs that are considered to be potentially damaging to their reproductive organs.

Drug abuse is only one aspect of women's behavior during pregnancy that can damage fetuses; smoking, drinking, and work place hazards are also considerations. If drug use during pregnancy is illegalized, are these restrictions on women's behavior far behind? What about the possibility of prosecuting diabetic women, or obese women, or women with cancer who need drugs that could harm the fetus, women with epilepsy, and women who are too poor to get the proper nutrition required for a healthy baby? These women should have the right to (a) decide to have children and accept the risks involved and (b) be free from criminal prosecution if something should happen to damage the fetus.

The potential implications of the criminalization of drug use during pregnancy are far-reaching: women's behavior could be monitored and regulated from the time that they menstruate, the moment they become able to bear children, through menopause, when they are no longer able to bear children. Infringements on the rights of all women are already in the works. Kansas State Representative Kerry Patrick introduced a bill that would require any convicted female drug addicts to have Norplant implanted if they want to avoid a jail sentence.[39] And, some companies have attempted to institute fetal protection policies that prohibit fertile women from holding jobs that entail exposure to harmful chemicals.

The case of Johnson Controls has received significant media attention over the last few years. Their policy bars fertile women from jobs that require lead exposure; according to Johnson's estimates this policy makes roughly half of their jobs unavailable to women. Johnson Controls and other corporations like Gulf Oil, B.F. Goodrich, DuPont, and Eastman Kodak, enacted these policies in order to avoid liability for the harmful

effects of their manufacturing processes on women and
fetuses; simply, they are trying to avoid having to pay
damages later. The Johnson Controls Policy has ignored
testimony of individual women regarding their
reproductive lives and their plans for childbearing; it
also ignores testimony stating that it is difficult to trace
birth defects to the effects of lead exposure, and
testimony that lead is equally harmful to the
reproductive systems of men. Why should women have
to pay for the effects of industrial production on
reproduction? In the same way that the criminal
prosecution of drug-using pregnant women diverts
resources that could be used to involve women in the
process of resolution, fetal protection policies exclude
women and attempt to free corporations of the
responsibility of eliminating the harmful effects of
production on its employees. Solving the problems will
cost the government and big businesses more than
covering them up will, however the differential should
not be taken out of women's paychecks or their
freedom.

The effect of fetal protection policies is to restrict the
number and type of jobs accessible to women in the
industrial workforce. The majority of the jobs that
would be off limits to women are highly unionized;
they are higher paying jobs with more opportunity for
advancement. Women cannot be expected to produce
healthy babies if they are denied access to the jobs that
afford them the opportunity to get care, treatment and
give them the opportunity to care for their children.

Recently the Supreme Court handed down its
decision in the case involving Johnson Controls. The
Court unequivocally upheld the rights of women to
employment: "fertile women may not be forced out of
their jobs to protect their unborn children." According
to Justice Blackmun, who also authored the 1973 *Roe*

opinion, "decisions about the welfare of future children must be left to the parents who conceive and raise them rather than to the employers who hire those parents."[40] This decision affirmed the rights of women to be free from discrimination on the basis of their childbearing capabilities. Fetal protection policies have been struck down because they violate a woman's right to equal protection and to privacy under the law.

The criminal prosecution of pregnant addicts amounts to discrimination on the basis of pregnancy. Policies that claim to protect women as reproductive units can lead to discrimination against them, as the Johnson Controls case illustrates, and to a violation of their constitutionally guaranteed rights. The acceptance of the criminal prosecution of women who use drugs during pregnancy into the mainstream threatens to limit the rights of women in this society. Women's unique capacity to bear children should not be viewed as reason enough to restrict women's access and freedom to the responsibilities and choices of life. They should not be relegated to childbearing vessels because society is unable to provide adequate care and treatment.

CONCLUSION

The use of criminal statutes to punish pregnant drug users cannot reduce the number of drug babies born each year. The program intimidates women to the point where they will not come forward for treatment knowing that they will be prosecuted. It denies that the inability of drug treatment programs to be able to accommodate the women sent into treatment by the criminal justice system exists. The political agenda needs to be reworked in such a way that priorities are reorganized and resources are redistributed. The prevalence of drug use among pregnant women coupled with the inaccessibility of care and treatment for most women leads to the deprioritization of women. When prosecutors then force the responsibility for these effects onto women, they are further disempowered. Women's status is lowered and respect for their well-being, let alone their rights, becomes secondary to those of the fetus. The main concern of those who object to the criminal prosecution of women who use drugs during pregnancy is that women will be required to relinquish more and more control as the campaign continues.

Women's rights advocates and civil libertarians warn against the slippery slope: if it is societally acceptable to make drug use during pregnancy equivalent to child abuse, if it is societally acceptable to exclude women from certain jobs simply because they are capable of bearing children, then is it acceptable to make it illegal to smoke cigarettes, drink alcohol, exercise, have sex, go to work, and travel during pregnancy, and will the state make an effort to regulate women's behavior to this extent in the name of fetal protection?

NOTES

[1] "Punishing Pregnant Addicts . . . " *New York Times*, 10 September 1989, IV, 5: 1.

[2] Ibid.

[3] National Association for Perinatal Addiction, Research and Education (NAPARE) "Update" October 1988.

[4] Ibid.

[5] "Beyond The Stereotypes: Women, Addiction and Perinatal Substance Abuse." Hearing before the Select Committee on Children, Youth and Families, House of Representatives, April 19, 1990, p. 4.

[6] Ibid, 7.

[7] Ibid, 15.

[8] Edmiston, 205.

[9] Michelle Oberman, "The Control of Pregnancy and the Criminalization of Femaleness," 7 *Berkeley Women's Law Journal* (1992): 9.

[10] Bonavoglia, 94.

[11] "Beyond the Stereotypes," 58.

[12] Gest, 67.

[13] Stephen Budiansky, "A Measure of Failure," *Atlantic Monthly*, January 1986, 32.

[14] Committee on Alcohol and Drug Dependent Women and Their Children, "Drug and Alcohol Related Issues and Pregnancy," State Legislative Briefing Book, 1991: 11-13.

[15] Nadine Brozan, "Close of Clinics Rocks Poor Women, " *New York Times*, 25 March 1991, A, 17.

[16] Robert Pear, "Spurning Bush, Congress provides New Money to Fight Infant Death, " *New York Times*, 26 March 1991, A, 21.

[17] "Beyond the Stereotypes," 588.

[18] Edmiston, 204.

[19] Wendy Chavkin, "Help, Don't Jail Addicted Mothers," *New York Times* ,18 July 1989, A, 22.

[20] Sachs, 105.

[21] LaCroix, 586.

[22] Paltrow, 44.

[23] Committee on Alcohol and Drug Dependent Women and Their Children, 10.

[24] Ibid.

[25] "Beyond the Stereotypes," 6.

[26] Committee on Alcohol and Drug Dependent Women and Their Children, 13.

[27] Ibid., 33.

[28] "Substance Abuse Treatment for Women: Crisis in Access," *Health Advocate*, Spring 1989, 9.

29 "Beyond the Stereotypes," 107-108.

30 Molly McNulty, "Combatting Pregnancy Discrimination
Access to Substance Abuse for Low-Income Women,"
Clearinghouse Review, May 1989, 22.

31 Committee on Alcohol and Drug Dependent Women and
Their Children, 12.

32 Wilkerson, 15.

33 Pollitt, 416.

34 Edmiston, 65.

35 Pollitt, 416.

36 Committee on Alcohol and Drug Dependent Women and
Their Children, 7.

37 Willwerth, 63.

38 Ibid.

39 Ibid.

40 Aaron Epstein, "High Court Extends Job Rights for
Women," *Miami Herald*, 21 March 1991, 1A.

Bibliography

Amana, Cheryl E., "Ethical and Legal Considerations of Maternal-Fetal Conflict in the Context of Substance Abuse." Master's Essay, Columbia University, School of Law, 1990.

American Civil Liberties Union. "State by State Case Summary of Criminal Prosecutions Against Pregnant Women," 29 October 1990.

American College of Obstetricians and Gynecologists, "Drug Abuse and Pregnancy," *Technical Bulletin* 96 (September 1986).

_____ "Patient Choice: Maternal-Fetal Conflict," *Committee Opinion* 55 (October 1987).

_____ "Cocaine Abuse: Implications for Pregnancy," *Committee Opinion* 81 (March 1990).

Begley, Sharon. "The Troubling Question of 'Fetal Rights.'" *Newsweek* (8 December 1986): 87-88.

Bonavoglia, Angela. "The Ordeal of Pamela Rae Stewart." *Ms.* (July/August 1987): 92-95+.

Bradley, Bill, Senator. "Healthy Birth Act of 1989," S. 708, 101st Congress, 1st session. 5 April 1989.

Brozan, Nadine, "Close of Clinics Rocks Poor Women," *New York Times*, 25 March 1991, A,17.

Budiansky, Stephen. "A Measure of Failure." *Atlantic Monthly* (January 1986): 32-33.

California Advocates for Pregnant Women, *Newsletter.* July/August 1990. (Their address is 2437 Second Avenue San Diego, CA 92101.)

Carey, Joseph with Jack A. Seamonds and Mary Galligan. "Infant Death Rate: Rise Linked to Health-Care Cuts." *U.S. News and World Report* (24 February 1986): 67-68.

Chavkin, Wendy, "Help, Don't Jail Addicted Mothers," *New York Times* 18 July 1989, A, 22.

Coalition on Alcohol and Drug Dependent Women and Their Children. "Drug and Alcohol Related Issues and Pregnancy." *State Legislative Briefing Book* (1991).

Crockett, Karen G. and Miriam Hyman. "Live Birth: A Condition Precedent to Recognition of Rights." *Hofstra Law Review* 4 (1976): 805-837.

Curriden, Mark. "Holding Mom Accountable." *ABA Journal* (March 1990): 51-53.

Edmiston, Susan. "Here Come the Pregnancy Police." *Glamour* (August 1990): 202-205+.

Epstein, Aaron, "High Court Extends Job Rights for Women," *Miami Herald*, 21 March 1991, A, 10.

Freitag, Michael, "Hospital Defends Limiting of Drug Program," *New York Times*, 12 October 1989, B, 9.

Gallagher, Janet. "Prenatal Invasions and Interventions: What's Wrong with Fetal Rights." *Harvard Women's Law Journal* 10 (1987): 9-38.

_____. "The Fetus and the Law--Whose Life Is It Anyway?" *Ms.* (September 1984): 63-66+.

Gest, Ted. "The Pregnancy Police on Patrol." *U.S. News and World Report* (6 February 1989): 50.

Hoffman, Jan. "Pregnant, Addicted--and Guilty?" *New York Times Magazine* (19 August 1990): 33-35+.

Johnsen, Dawn E. "The Creation of Fetal Rights: Conflicts with Women's Constitutional Rights to Liberty, Privacy, and Equal Protection." *Yale Law Journal* 95 (1986): 599-625.

Jost, Kenneth. "Mother Versus Child." *Law and Medicine* (April 1989): 84-89.

"Judge Drops Charges of Delivering Drugs To an Unborn Baby," *New York Times,* 5 February 1991, 6: 4.

Kolder, Veronika E. B., Janet Gallagher, and Michael T. Parsons. "Court-Ordered Obstetrical Interventions." *The New England Journal Of Medicine* (7 May 1987): 1192-1196.

Lacayo, Richard. "Do the Unborn Have Rights?" *Time* (Fall 1990): 22-23.

LaCroix, Susan. "Jailing Mothers for Drug Abuse." *The Nation* (1 May 1989): 585-588.

Lewin, Tamar, "Court in Florida Upholds Conviction For Drug Delivery by Umbilical Cord," *New York Times*, 20 April, 1991, I, 6: 4.

_____. "When Courts Take Charge of the Unborn," *New York Times*, 9 January 1989, I, 1: 1.

Losco, Joseph. "Fetal Abuse: an Exploration of Emerging Philosophic, Legal, and Policy Issues." *Western Political Quarterly* (June 1989): 265-286.

Marcus, Dockser and Amy Stevens, "Michigan Woman Won't be Tried for Delivering Drugs to Her Fetus," *Wall Street Journal*, n.d., n.p.

McNulty, Molly. "Combating Pregnancy Discrimination in Access to Substance Abuse Treatment for Low-Income Women." *Clearinghouse Review* (May 1989): 21-25.

_____. "Pregnancy Police: The Health Policy and Legal Implications of Punishing Pregnant Women for Harm to their Fetuses." *New York University Review of Law and Social Change* 19 (1987-88): 277-319.

"Michigan Court Backs Mother in Drug Case," *New York Times*, 18 July, 1991, B, 7: 2.

Moss, Kary L. "Legal Issues: Drug Testing of Postpartum Women and Newborns as the Basis for Civil and Criminal Proceedings." *Clearinghouse Review* (March 1990): 1406-1414.

Myers, R. "Abuse and Neglect of the Unborn." *Duquesne Law Review* 23 (1984): 4-64.

National Association for Perinatal Addiction Research and Education, *Update.* October 1988.

Oberman, Michelle. "The Control of Pregnancy and the Criminalization of Femaleness." 7 *Berkeley Women's Law Journal* (1992): 1-12.

Paltrow, Lynn M. "When Becoming Pregnant is a Crime." *Criminal Justice Ethics* (Winter/Spring 1990): 41-47.

Pear, Robert, "Spurning Bush, Congress Provides New Money to Fight Infant Death," *New York Times*, 26 March 1991, A, 1.

Pollitt, Katha. "A New Assault on Feminism." *The Nation* (26 March 1990): 409-418.

"Punishing Pregnant Addicts: Debate, Destiny, No Solution," *New York Times*, 10 September 1989, IV, 5: 1.

Roberts, Dorothy E. "The Future of Reproductive Choice for Poor Women and Women of Color." *Women's Rights Law Reporter* (Summer 1990): 66-69.

_____. "Mother as Martyr." *Essence* (May 1991): 140.

Robertson. "Procreative Liberty and the Control of Conception, Pregnancy, and Childbirth." *Virginia Law Review* 69 (1983): 405-438.

Sachs, Andrea. "Here Come the Pregnancy Police." *Time* (22 May 1989): 104-105.

Stone, Deborah A. "Fetal Risks, Women's Rights." *The American Prospect* (Fall 1990): 43-53.

"Substance Abuse Treatment for Women: Crisis in Access." *Health Advocate* 160 (Spring 1989): 9-10.

"Suit Seeks Drug Treatment for Pregnant Women," *New York Times*, 10 December 1989, I, 62: 1.

U.S. Congress. House Select Committee on Children, Youth, and Families. *Beyond the Stereotypes: Women, Addiction, and Perinatal Substance Abuse.* 101st Congress, second session, 1990.

Westfall. "Beyond Abortion: the Potential Reach of the Human Life Amendment." *Defining Human Life: Medical, Legal, and Ethical Implications.* Marjery Shaw and A. Edward Doudera, eds. (AUPHA Press, 1983).

Willwerth, James. "Should We Take Away Their Kids?" *Time* (13 May 1991): 62-63.

Wilkerson, Isabel, "Woman Cleared After Drug Use in Pregnancy," *New York Times*, 3 April 1991, A, 15.

Wilson, Pete, Senator. "Child Abuse During Pregnancy Prevention Act of 1989," S. 1444, 101st Congress, 1st session. 31 July 1989.

Index